Research Methods and Statistics in Health Care

The book is dedicated with love and thanks
to our mothers
Sarah Glasgow Reid
and
Bronwen Mills Boore

Research Methods and Statistics in Health Care

Norma G. Reid BSc, MSc, DPhil, FSS
Director
Centre for Applied Health Studies
University of Ulster at Coleraine

Jennifer R. P. Boore SRN, SCM, PhD, RNT
Professor
Department of Nursing and Health Visiting
University of Ulster at Coleraine

Edward Arnold

© Norma J. Reid and Jennifer R. P. Boore 1987

First published in Great Britain 1987 by
Edward Arnold (Publishers) Ltd, 41 Bedford Square, London WC1B 3DQ

Edward Arnold (Australia) Pty Ltd, 80 Waverley Road, Caulfield East,
Victoria 3145, Australia

Edward Arnold, 3 East Read Street, Baltimore, Maryland 21202, U.S.A.

British Library Cataloguing in Publication Data

Reid, Norma G.
    Research methods and statistics in health care.
    1. Medicine——Research
    I. Title   II. Boore, Jennifer R.P.
    610'.72   R852

    ISBN 0-7131-4522-6

Text set in 10/11 pt Plantin
by Colset Private Limited, Singapore
Made and printed in Great Britain
by Richard Clay plc, Bungay, Suffolk

Preface

This book has been written for the practising nurse. It is also suitable for other health care professions. It begins by addressing the role and usefulness of research methods and statistics in such professions, and then provides an introduction to research methods in Chapters 2 and 3 and a step by step account of basic statistical techniques in Chapters 4, 5 and 6. The final chapter provides three practical examples illustrating the value of these techniques and methods.

Those who master the contents of this book will find that they have acquired skills which should enhance their professional performance. This in turn should result in better care for the patients and clients we serve.

1987

N. G. R.
J. R. P. B.

Acknowledgement

The publishers would like to thank Faber & Faber and Random House Inc for 'The Unknown Citizen' and part of 'Under which Lyre' from *W H Auden: Collected Poems* edited by Mendelson © 1946.

Contents

1

Research Methods and Statistics in Nursing:

The Social, Professional and Cultural Context

'To understand God's thoughts we must study statistics, for these are the measure of His purpose' *Florence Nightingale* (1820–1910)   (Pearson, 1924)

Introduction

The suggestion of divine endorsement for the study of statistics is likely to provide grounds for doubts in the sturdiest believer, but this quotation is further remarkable for being one of few positive statements on record about the subject of statistics. Still less worldly acclaim has come the way of those who practise statistics. The professional statistician occupies a place in the ladder of the public's affections just one step up from traffic wardens, and one step down from the taxman. In the unlikely event that the public's attitude to statistics and statisticians were ever thought a topic of sufficient interest or importance to warrant an opinion poll, we should no doubt find the subject perceived as dull, devious and downright dangerous, whilst its perpetrators would be classed as professionally unreliable and socially undesirable.

The image of the researcher is probably a little more up-market and considerably less unpleasant, but it is likely that few people see researchers as essential to the common good or integral to the world at large. A certain glamour still attaches to the traditional image of the boffin intent on his manuscripts or microscopes in his ivory tower, but this is nowadays offset by the more common manifestation of the researcher banging on the doors of County Hall or ICI, desperately seeking a few pieces of gold to allow him to pursue his essential and valuable work. Whether he is an absent-minded professor or a struggling greenhorn on a fixed-term contract, he will be perceived as a less than effective communicator, who is a mile or two removed from reality and somewhat distanced from the workaday concerns of ordinary people.

It is no surprise therefore that the public feel neither excitement about, nor empathy with, the study of statistics or research. Still less do the health professions whose business it is to care and nurture and heal. Those whose concern is with the quality of life are less inclined than most to espouse the science of numbers and then crunch them. Yet the training for these same professions increasingly requires compulsory doses of research methods and statistics. The process – which has been likened to a nasogastric tube feed – causes consternation in both the teachers and the taught. These same professions are also showing alarming tendencies to incorporate the wiles of the statistician and researcher into everyday practice. Nursing has been charged to be a research based profession. Computers are sprouting on hospital wards and some fear they will soon displace the patients in the beds, the staff having long since become redundant. Nurse managers grapple more often with t-tests than teacups, and tutors in their lunch breaks discuss Likert scales and salary scales with equal animation.

So what has all of this to do with caring? The traditional image of the nurse soothing the fevered brow and comforting the sufferer with soft words is revered in our society and rightly so. But nowadays the nurse will be as likely as not concurrently assessing, monitoring, educating, evaluating, calibrating (and probably fulminating) – and simultaneously recording the results on a 23 page questionnaire. It is worth asking whether all of this is possible, but more important perhaps to ask why it is being done and whether the best use is being made of the information which is being recorded.

In any profession, the filling out of endless forms and the routine recording of information is regarded as perhaps tedious, but nonetheless an inescapable activity. Yet there is often considerable frustration about the necessity for so much clerical work, and questions are raised about the usefulness of the information recorded. Nurses, for example, in a normal working day will fill in the kardex, bed state forms, off-duty rotas, patient admission forms, discharge forms, transfer forms, fluid balance sheets, records of temperature, pulse and respiration rates and blood pressures, and nursing process forms. It will not be unusual for a ward to be additionally involved in providing documentation for staffing establishment methods like the Telford method, the Cheltenham method, quality of care measures such as MONITOR or GRASP, or a dependency study, or a nurse hours per patient study.

The information recorded daily by nurses could be classified into three categories: patient related clinical information essential to the daily care of each patient, research related information, and administrative information about the workload and resources of the ward. A more detailed look at each of these categories may be useful.

Clinical information

The recording of clinical information about each patient is probably the most easily justified. Even here, however, questions can be asked about its necessity. It is by no means thought necessary in other countries, and even in all parts of the UK, to take and record temperature, pulse and blood pressure twice daily or four hourly for every patient. It could be argued that, even when this is not essential, it provides structured contact with the patient and is an opportunity for the nurse to talk to the patient and for the patient to make contact with the nurse. Do we need 'excuses' for such patient contact? Is it all that easy for a patient to generate a conversation with a nurse who has a stethoscope in her ears, or who is intent on counting a pulse rate? Many would argue that a proportion of these routine clinical observations serve no useful clinical or social purpose, and are therefore time consuming and play their part in generating vast mounds of paper.

The taking of routine observations illustrates readily, however, the implicit role of statistical ideas in nursing. Almost always the observation is classified as normal or abnormal. This is done either on the basis of well known norms, or of past experience. In either case these norms are estimates of the means of the relevant distributions. For example, the normal temperature for adults is 37°C and the normal blood pressure is 120/80. For particular age groups, sexes or other characteristics, these norms are understood to vary a little. When a temperature or a blood pressure differs from the norm by a certain amount, it is denoted abnormal. This implicitly uses the notion of a standard deviation (see page 65). The statistician would often define abnormality as lying more than two standard deviations from the mean. The nurse in practice is doing something very similar in identifying an observation as abnormal.

A good deal of routine nursing is therefore based on numerical measurements and the interpretation of these. Whether or not the nurse is explicitly aware of the statistical nature of this exercise, there is no doubt that statistical processes are present and it may well be that greater understanding of these processes would be helpful to the practice of nursing.

Diagnosis is another common activity which is underpinned by statistical ideas. When a patient is admitted to a diagnostic category, this is done on the basis of past knowledge or experience about the relationship between symptoms and a particular disease or condition. For example, a patient exhibiting symptoms of severe chest or back pains and breathlessness might well be diagnosed as having had a pulmonary embolism. This is because these symptoms have in the past been shown to be those of sufferers from pulmonary embolism. It is possible, of course, that the correct diagnosis may be quite different, but past experience has shown that other diagnoses are less likely to be correct. The assignment to a diagnostic category is, therefore, based on a balance of probabilities. As more examinations and tests are done, more information becomes available and at some point a diagnosis will become certain.

The pioneering work of de Dombal and his colleagues in computers and medicine (de Dombal *et al.*, 1974) demonstrated the contribution of the computer in such a context. The human diagnostician makes a judgment on the basis of his data bank – his memory and knowledge. The size and quality of this data bank will depend on the amount of his experience, his capacity to retain and organise information, the correctness of his judgements about that information, and a whole set of human and personal factors. The computer can also make a diagnosis, if the relevant information is fed into its memory. The computer has one immediate advantage in that its memory is perfect and its consciousness unclogged by any extraneous concerns like the car needing new tyres or the children being ill. The work of de Dombal and his colleagues showed that computer diagnosis on the basis of a data base derived from information gathered over a five year period, was a little better than that of the most experienced consultant and markedly better than that of more junior medical staff. The computer worked explicitly on calculating the probabilities of specific diagnoses based on past experience – and the computer got these absolutely correct. The human diagnostician implicitly uses the same process, but constrained by a limited memory bank and ordinary human weaknesses. We emphasise that we are not recommending the replacement of human carers with computers, but are highlighting the extent to which considerable sections of the processes carried out by humans are based on statistical ideas, and have been shown to be replicable using technology which is now available.

Research related information

The second category of information routinely collected and recorded on wards is related to research. This is often initiated by senior nursing staff in collaboration with outside researchers. Particular emphasis has recently been placed on methods which attempt to establish staffing levels, some of which were listed earlier in this chapter. The information required for these exercises can be tedious and time consuming to record at ward level. The impression is that staff at ward level often do not know much about these methods or why it is important to carry out such studies. Staff also are often heard to say that they 'never get anything back from research'.

The first problem to be tackled here is the perception of research as something apart. The onus is on the researchers with the senior nursing staff to explain why research studies are useful and important. Secondly, it is important that ward staff should ask for and insist on a full explanation before collecting information, and a promise of feedback afterwards. Those who provide information have a right to receive information back. It is often the case that information collected as part of a research study will have a local usefulness and relevance beyond the remit of the study.

Some years ago a study of nurse training in the clinical area was carried out in Northern Ireland (Reid, 1986). As part of this study, a patient dependency study was carried out with a view to calculating and comparing workloads across the study wards. For each ward a profile of its workload was produced over a sixty day period. The ward sisters were put to considerable trouble in keeping records on a daily basis so, in return, each ward was sent its own profile, with some summary figures on workload and the average figures for the hospital, district and area. In one hospital, two adjacent and structurally identical medical wards had been included. The results of this dependency study showed that the female medical ward had on average twice the workload of the male medical ward, yet the levels of staffing were almost identical. The ward sister on the female medical ward had been trying for some time to make the case for more staff, without result. Within a short time of this research evidence being received, however, she was allocated the extra staff. This illustrates the usefulness of well collated and well presented information in influencing decisions. This particular information was collected for a specific purpose within a research study, but had further local value when fed back to the staff who produced it.

Nurses and other health care professionals should be urged to co-operate in research studies, but to insist on feedback and to use that feedback constructively in investigating local issues.

This leads into the third category of information gathering which is to do with administration and management.

Administrative information

Typical examples of such information would be off-duty rotas and bed state forms. The potential of these humble routine forms for the planning and management of care is vastly underestimated by nurses themselves. A set of off-duty rotas contains invaluable information about, for example, the mix of skills available to wards in different periods of the day and night, the ratio of trained staff to others, the ratio of trained staff to learners and levels of support by nursing auxiliaries. It is very rare that analyses are carried out to elicit such information. If computers were used to develop and produce off-duty rotas it would be a simple matter to programme them to obtain routine print-outs of all the above factors and many more. Within a hospital this would be an enormous help to unit managers in monitoring resources across wards.

Bed state forms can be, and often are, analysed to produce indices of patient turnover, bed occupancy and throughput for a ward. This is rarely done at ward level however, being most commonly a task for the medical records department, and the information is even more rarely relayed back to those who plan and deliver care.

Recent research studies in Northern Ireland (e.g. Reid and Melaugh, 1987) have been based solely on the information available from off-duty rotas and bed state forms. This work could be done by any nurse. It involves the calculation of a ratio for each day: the number of nursing hours (from the off-duty rota) divided by the number of occupied beds. This index, called the NHPP ratio (nursing hours per patient) can be calculated each day and over a month, and might show enormous fluctuations within a ward, or enormous differences between one ward and another of a similar type. There may be reasons for this. It may be very sensible and desirable to have more nursing hours per patient on theatre days, or intake days, or the difference in patient dependency from one ward to another may justify different levels of nurse hours per patient. Yet it has been found in studies covering hundreds of wards that differences in staffing can rarely be explained or justified. In most cases, the levels of staffing have arisen historically and pragmatically and are not related to actual patient load.

How to use this information
The collation of routinely available information has therefore a very considerable untapped potential in the planning and management of care. This collation and summarisation of information requires basic statistical skills, well within the grasp of any qualified nurse. These skills are essential in the modern world, not least because in periods of shrinking resources we must be able to justify and defend the resources we have. This means that it is necessary to have the ability to use figures to support a case, and to use them effectively. No one wants to read pages covered with numbers. What is required is a summary of these numbers. Yet how many nurses have learnt how to reduce a page of numbers to two or three summary numbers which convey almost as much information? This book deals with these basic and practical skills in numeracy, which do not require a doctorate in mathematics, or even an 'A' level. All of these techniques have been successfully taught to a variety of professional groups some of whose members did not even have 'O' level mathematics.

Value of research methods

The book also encompasses research methods, but at a very practical level. Research should not be an elevated and highly technical business conducted by academics in isolation from the world. Research methods can and should be part of every professional's toolbox of skills. For research methods, at their most basic, provide no more than a logical approach to problem solving. We believe that research should be carried out with collaboration between academics and professionals, but would stress that there is no reason why practising nurses should not themselves employ a research based approach to problem solving. This approach will simply identify and clearly state the problem, collect the relevant information and analyse it. This book helps in the detail of what is involved, provides some help on the basic techniques (like questionnaire design) and offers a simple but practical range of statistical techniques which can be used in the analysis of information.

The questions which can be addressed using a research framework can be related in a very immediate way to patient care. A nurse may, for example, have noticed that patients who are well prepared for the experience of an operation tend to have a better experience of recovery and tend to develop fewer post-operative complications. She may strongly suspect that this is so, but may wish to establish her case in an objective way with a view to influencing the practice of others. In fact this question is a large scale research exercise and has been the subject of doctoral theses (Boore, 1978; Hayward, 1975), but it could be explored in a small scale study on one ward, provided it was done in a structured way and the limitations were recognised. It would involve a careful definition of the preparation process, the selection of patients for a research programme (and the selection of similar patients to compare with those on the programme), and carefully structured recording of events before and after the operation. So research techniques can and should be part of the normal working life of those who work in the health professions.

There is a story about a man who wanted to buy a donkey, but was concerned about the cruelty involved in the training of donkeys. So he was delighted to see an advertisement in a local paper offering for sale donkeys trained through kind and humane methods. He went to meet the dealer, who confirmed that the donkeys were trained to respond to humane treatment; that they had only to be instructed quietly and kindly and they would obey any order. The man took his donkey home but the following weeks were full of frustration, for all his calm and kindly requests were ignored by the donkey who just stood there munching grass. Eventually he took the donkey back to the dealer and explained the problem. The dealer lifted a shovel and hit the donkey an enormous whack over the ear. 'What are you doing?' cried the humanitarian, 'I thought you said the donkey was trained to respond only to kindness.' 'Ah yes,' said the dealer, 'so it is. But first you have to get its attention!'

A foray into the world of statistics and research methods can feel to many health care professionals like a whack on the ear with a shovel. But we assure you that as far as possible our methods in this book will be humane. We are not in the business of making health professionals into statisticians or researchers – there are more than enough of those already! But we do believe that the readers of this book will find that the skills we aim to help them develop will enhance their performance as caring professionals, and in the longer term will benefit the organization, management and delivery of care, which is the core of what we are all trying to do.

The historical and cultural context

Before diving cheerily into mounds of formulae and algebra, it is helpful to understand the historical and cultural context of statistics and research methods in the health care professions. These issues are addressed in a way which will hopefully both explain the alienation many feel to these subjects, and also underline their importance.

Many nurses and other health workers feel nowadays that statistics have been foisted upon them. The truth is rather different, for the most famous nurse of all time, Florence Nightingale, was a pioneer of the study of statistics and one of the earliest advocates of the subject. Known as 'the passionate statistician' she believed statistics to be 'the most important science in the whole world'.

Florence Nightingale was a reformer. Through her work in the Crimea and later in England she recognised that to tackle the appalling death rates from preventable diseases and to achieve effective reform a logical approach was needed, based on systematic gathering and analysis of information.

She was acquainted with many of the intellectuals of her time. In fact her friendship with Sir Edwin Chadwick, the pioneer of the public health movement, considerably predated her Crimean work and Chadwick was a great source of influence and encouragement to the young Florence Nightingale.

On her return from the Crimea, Florence Nightingale began a campaign aimed at producing reform in both the army and in the hospitals. She

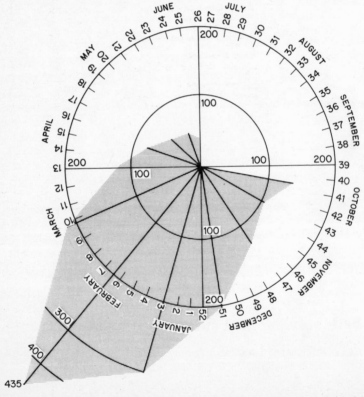

Fig. 1.1 Florence Nightingale's diagram illustrating mortality rate at Scutari (the main British hospital in the Crimean War) in the winter of 1854–55. Sanitary reforms, largely influenced by Nightingale, began in March and, as depicted here, there was subsequently a sharp decline in the death rate.

designed 'model forms' for the recording of disease classifications and, through her friend Dr William Farr, a physician and professional statistician, had this form discussed at an International Statistical Congress held in 1860 in London. Her model forms (called 'Miss Nightingale's scheme for Uniform Hospital Statistics') were well received and adopted at once by a number of the prestigious London hospitals.

The years between the end of the Crimean War and 1860 were filled with activity. Florence Nightingale lobbied and wrote prolifically. Of particular interest is her use of statistical diagrams to strengthen her case. She had begun to produce such diagrams in the Crimea and indeed she claimed to have invented the use of pictorial diagrams.

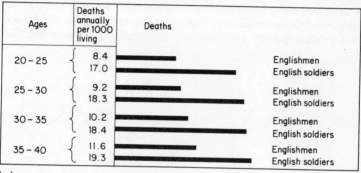

(a)

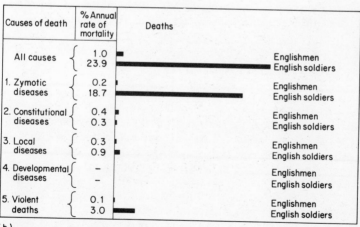

(b)

Fig. 1.2 Line diagrams from the Royal Commission's report (1858) comparing conditions in the army to those in civilian life. (**a**) The relative mortality of the peace-time army and male population in Britain at corresponding ages. (**b**) The relative mortality, from various causes, of the army in hospital during the Crimean War and of the English male population, aged 15–45.

The polar area diagram was invented by Florence Nightingale and she called such diagrams 'coxcombs'.

Her campaign using such evidence was influential in causing a Royal Commission on the Health of the Army to be set up in 1858. Although it was not possible for a woman at that time to serve on such a board, Florence Nightingale provided a mass of evidence to the board and influenced its deliberations through friends like Chadwick who were members. She even had the statistical section of the Report reprinted at her own expense and distributed it widely in Parliament and among friends. Line diagrams from the Report of the Royal Commission (1858) further illustrate Nightingale's innovative approach to representation of statistics (Fig. 1.2).

Her interest in statistics continued throughout her life and she was particularly fascinated by Quételet, the Belgian mathematician. They met several times and shared a conviction that the study of statistics was the key to the moral and spiritual universe – what Quételet called 'the laws of moral statistics'. She was shattered by Quételet's death in 1874 and tried to have his work republished after his death.

She was opposed to pure theory, and the dichotomy between theoretical and practical statistics is illustrated by an interesting incident involving Florence Nightingale and Sir Francis Galton, the most eminent statistician of the time. She initially left £2000 in her will to endow the first ever university chair of applied statistics in the UK. Galton, however, refused to exclude research from the endowment, as Nightingale wished (her intention being to promote educational work in the *use* of statistics), so she revoked the bequest in her will.

It is ironic that many modern nurses are resistant to the use of statistics when the founder of modern nursing was one of its greatest advocates.

Attitudes towards statistics

A dislike and distrust of statistics runs very deep in our culture. The term statistics has two meanings; it can refer to the practice of collecting numerical data, but also to the practice of making inferences from that data. The latter is a relatively recent discipline, but the collection of statistics can be traced back to the Roman Empire in the well known census of Caesar Augustus. It is likely, however, that counting people was practised very much earlier than this, usually to assess numbers available for military duty or taxation. There are in fact old Testament references to a census in the Book of Numbers.

The first use of statistics as an analytical tool is ascribed to John Graunt (1620–1674), author of early writing on the subject. Graunt collected data on plague deaths in 1603 and from these made estimates of the population of London. He was the first to produce the idea of representative sampling as a basis for inference to a bigger population. Through the next two centuries the enumeration of vital statistics grew steadily and by the end of the nineteenth century the collection and analysis of data were widespread. The growth of what is now called social science occurred in the same period, and it is of interest to note how the history of statistics has been linked to various social movements, particularly in the nineteenth century. This involved statistics with some movements which are, with hindsight, less than desirable and may account in part for modern antipathy to the subject.

In particular the eugenics movement attracted some of the great names in statistics in the late nineteenth and twentieth century. First Galton and then Karl Pearson and R. A. Fisher, the greatest statisticians of their respective times, were deeply involved in eugenics. The eugenicists believed that standards of health, social behaviour and intelligence could be raised by selective breeding. The empirical basis of much of their work lay in probability theory. In its early years this movement was associated with Darwinian ideas and, to be fair to those involved, did not have the very undesirable connotations later attached to eugenics through its adoption by the fascist movements of Europe. Through the involvement of statisticians with eugenics many of the great classical statistical theories are published in, for example, *The Annals of Eugenics*. Nowadays, for good reasons, we are deeply antipathetic to eugenics and related philosophies. It would be interesting to know the extent to which the public are aware of the historical link between statistics and eugenics and whether this contributes to a fear and distrust of statistics in our culture.

There are many famous quotes about statistics and statisticians and an analysis of those which appear in dictionaries of quotations (*Concise Oxford Dictionary of Quotations*, 1982) reveals that two themes recur; first, that statistics are cold, uncaring and inhuman, and second that statistics lie and bewilder.

The theme of statistics being uncaring is well illustrated by a quote from David Lloyd George (1863–1945) who said that 'you cannot feed the hungry on statistics'. A rather unlikelier political comment on the implications of statistics came from Stalin (1879–1953) who wrote 'a single death is a tragedy, a million deaths is a statistic'.

It is easy to understand why the reduction or representation of human misery to numbers and statistics seems inhumane and heartless. But many commentators have considered any collection of statistics on human beings to be offensive. George Markstein and David Tomblin both stated 'I am not a number – I am a free man'.

Dickens (1812–1870) satirised the role of statistics and statisticians in a number of his books, most notably in *Hard Times*. The poet, W. H. Auden (1907–1973) had a particular contempt for both statistics and social sciences and in several of his poems employed his cutting wit at their expense. For example, *Under which Lyre*, a Reactionary Tract for the Times includes:

> Thou shalt not sit with statisticians
> nor commit a Social Science.

and: Out of the air, a voice without a face
                        Proved by statistics that some cause was just
                        In tones as dry and level as the place.

It was in his poem *The Unknown Citizen* (to JS/07/M/378 this Marble
Monument is erected by the State) that Auden developed his dislike of social
science and statisticians and linked their activities to those of Orwell's
futuristic *1984* type state which collects endless statistics on its citizens, but
cares little for the fundamental individual human conditions of freedom and
happiness. The poem is worth quoting in full as a splendid example of the
reasons why statistics is held to be a cold and uncaring subject.

He was as found by the Bureau of Statistics to be
One against whom there was no official complaint,
And all the reports on his conduct agree
That, in the modern sense of an old-fashioned word, he was a saint,
For in everything he did he served the Greater Community.
Except for the War till the day he retired
He worked in a factory and never got fired,
But satisfied his employers, Fudge Motors Inc.
Yet he wasn't a scab or odd in his views,
For his Union reports that he paid his dues,
(Our Report on his Union shows it was sound)
And our Social Psychology workers found
That he was popular with his mates and liked a drink.
The Press are convinced that he bought a paper every day
And that his reactions to advertisements were normal in every way.
Policies taken out in his name prove that he was fully insured,
And his Health-card shows he was once in hospital but left it cured.
Both Producers Research and High-Grade Living declare
He was fully sensible to the advantages of the Instalment Plan
And had everything necessary to the Modern Man,
A phonograph, a radio, a car and a frigidaire.
Our researchers into Public Opinion are content
That he held the proper opinions for the time of year;
When there was peace, he was for peace; when there was war, he went.
He was married and added five children to the population,
Which our Eugenist says was the right number for a parent of his
generation,
And our teachers report that he never interfered with their education.
Was he free? Was he happy? The question is absurd:
Had anything been wrong, we should certainly have heard.

The charge that statistics lie is embodied in the well known quote
attributed to Mark Twain: 'There are three kinds of lies – lies, damned lies
and statistics', a quote which became famous after it was used by Disraeli

(1804–1881) in the House of Commons. Many other examples of this theme can be found in most dictionaries of quotations. For example,

There are two kinds of statistics, the kind you look up and the kind you make up. *Rex Stout*

You may prove anything by figures. *Thomas Carlyle*

Statistics are like alienists – they will testify for either side.
F. H. La Guardia

In modern life the manipulation of statistics has unfortunately become a routine part of advertising and public relations. Election times provide a plethora of examples of how to manipulate (wrongly) statistics to support or prove your point. Darrell Huff (1954) in his book *How to Lie with Statistics* provides a readable account of the ways in which basic statistics are misused and this book is recommended to those who need to interpret statistics in their professional roles.

So how do we respond to the charges that statistics is an uncaring and untruthful subject? On the former point, we believe, like Florence Nightingale, that statistics are an essential part of the toolkit of a caring professional. Statistics are not of themselves important, but they can help us to identify, understand and interpret the world of the caring professional and thus to enhance the quality of the care we provide. To the charge that statistics lie, we respond that it is not statistics which lie, but those who misuse statistics either in ignorance or with intent to manipulate. Statistics are neutral, those who use them are not. The intention of this book is to provide a basic grounding in statistics and it is our hope that it will help the reader to distinguish between the spurious and the genuine statistic. We cannot do better than commend Thomas Carlyle's (1795–1881) dictum that 'A judicious man . . . looks at statistics, not to get knowledge, but to save himself from having ignorance foisted on him.'

Nursing is developing into a research based profession and statistics play an important part in the examination and interpretation of the results of the research. The next two chapters look fairly briefly at the research process and some of the methods that practising nurses may use in the examination of problems in their everyday work. The majority of this book, however, examines methods of dealing with the data thus collected.

2

The Research Process

The term 'research' means different things to different people. To the professional researcher it can mean large scale studies lasting for several years with a team of full-time purpose-appointed staff and full technological back-up. To others 'research' can be simply looking into something in a bit more depth – 'I did a bit of research into that a few years back'. Whatever the scale of the research project, it is suggested that worthwhile research is characterised by a logical approach to solving a problem or obtaining and analysing information. This logical approach is called the research process.

There are a number of distinct stages in the research process, although some may occur in parallel.

Selection and formulation of a research problem, including reviewing relevant literature
Stating the aims and objectives of the research
Design of the study and choice of methods
Funding
Ethical considerations
Communications
Construction of instruments
Pilot study
Data collection
Analysis
Presentation of Findings

Each of these stages are examined in some detail.

Selection and formulation of a research problem

A research problem can arise in two ways; it can come to you or you can look for it. It may be that in the course of work as a nurse some issue arises which would be amenable to investigation through research. This might be a development in nursing practice or a response to a problem such as absenteeism. Whatever the nature of the issue, it is something which arises naturally from professional practice. Alternatively you may for some reason wish to or be required to carry out a research project. You may have joined a research appreciation course or be studying for an educational qualification where a small research project is required.

At this early stage the research area of interest is likely to be very general. For example, post operative care or attitudes to full student status for learners or the adequacy of basic training in providing management skills might be typical broad areas of interest. Even at this early stage it is worth considering your resources for research before proceeding further.

In considering the resources available a number of questions need to be asked. How much time do you have? Have you any funding to cover the costs of collecting data? Have you access to any secretarial support for typing and clerical work? Have you helpers for the data collection? How will you analyse the results? Have you access to a computer or will analysis be done with only the help of a pocket calculator?

If you have only a couple of months of your own time and no extra human or financial support, you should plan a very small scale study indeed. Allow perhaps a month for the design of your study, a couple of weeks for data collection and a month for analysis and report writing. This seems to be an absolute minimum time-scale even for the smallest project.

Let us look further at the example research area of attitudes to full student status for learners, on the assumption that you have 2–3 months and minimum resources. Your lack of time and resources might suggest that a postal survey would be the best approach, being relatively cheap. But where can you obtain a sampling frame of names and addresses and on what scale should the project be? To cover the whole of the UK is clearly out of the question. The best source of addresses would probably be the DHSS (England and Wales), the DHSS (Northern Ireland) and the Scottish Home and Health Department. But the obtaining of access to this information might well be refused (government has to be very careful on confidentiality of names and addresses, and the Data Protection Act has placed additional constraints on the release of information held on computer) and in any case the negotiation for such information could take several months with no guarantee of a successful outcome. So it would seem that the study could only be carried out on a more local level. You could perhaps survey a sample of nursing staff in your own hospital if your senior nursing officer will make names and addresses available to you. You have now redefined the research area from a study of attitudes to student status to a study of attitudes in one hospital to student status.

At this point it may be necessary to give further thought to a definition of student status. This is interpreted in a variety of ways. The researcher must be absolutely clear about what is meant by such terms and to communicate this clearly to those who participate in the study.

The next question is 'whose attitudes?' Are you going to survey all qualified staff or only registered nurses: are you going to include learners in the study? You feel that it is the attitude of qualified registered staff which is of most importance. You have now redefined the study once more to a survey of attitudes of registered nurses in one hospital to student status.

It is this process of honing down the research area to a specific research statement which is the important initial step in research. Almost always the problem as originally stated will be too broad. There are two other important activities associated with formulation of a research question.

Review of the literature and consulting experts

The first is a review of published research on the topic. There is no point in re-inventing the wheel. Someone else may already have tackled and solved your problem. The second is to identify any person local to you who might be able to advise you in formulating the problem – and indeed in where to begin your literature review. It is worth trying to identify and form links with any person or institution in your locality which might be helpful in your research. There may be a polytechnic or a university with a department of nursing or with active health researchers. There may be a school or college of nursing with a good library and a senior tutor particularly interested in research. Most researchers in higher education will be sympathetic and helpful if asked for a brief consultation. Most tutors with a research interest are only too glad to help a fellow professional to initiate some research.

The literature search can be begun by first checking the list of nursing journals available in a library and selecting the likeliest ones on the basis of the title. You can then go through back numbers, initially just looking at the lists of papers and reading the useful ones. Once a recent useful paper has been found, the references in it will allow earlier references to be traced backwards in time. However, a helpful professional researcher may be able to save you time by providing some references as a starting point.

Two important publications of value in searching the nursing literature are the *International Nursing Index* (published by the American Journal of Nursing Co.) and the *RCN Bibliography* (published by the Royal College of Nursing). These allow you to look up key words about your study area and find out what has been published in the journals surveyed by the publication. The *International Nursing Index* covers a very wide range of nursing journals, while the *RCN Bibliography* covers fewer journals but is published more frequently (monthly) and is therefore more up-to-date and also includes some books. Articles which appear highly relevant from their titles and are not available in your local library may be obtained through inter-library loan, if you have access to this service, or from the Royal College of Nursing Library in London who will send articles by post to their members.

The modern technological aid in literature searches is the computer search. In response to a few key words specified by you, (e.g. post-operative nursing care) the computer will search for all relevant publications in the major journals and provide you with a list of references. It is important to specify several key words, otherwise the computer will produce thousands of references – in response to 'nursing, education' for example! You can probably pay for a computer search in most university libraries – the cost is usually £20–30.

Once the literature has been reviewed by technological or more mundane means, you can see where your proposed study fits. Has it been done? Perhaps it was done in another country and you could replicate the study on your home ground. Or perhaps a similar study was done for another grade of nurse and you could adapt it for the grade you want to study. You will probably be stimulated by the research of others to develop your own. If another researcher has developed a good questionnaire which meets your needs, use it. You must, of course, write to the researcher and ask permission. Normally permission is granted willingly provided full acknowledgement is given.

So through the process of reading the literature, asking yourself a number of searching questions and discussing your research with others, the research problem will become increasingly defined and clear. You should indeed be beginning to develop a feel for the methods that might be appropriate. The end point of this initial stage is to be able to write down a concise short statement of the research problem.

Research problem: To explore the attitudes of a sample of registered nurses in one hospital to student status for nurse learners.

Aims and objectives of the research

It is probably helpful to consider now the aims and objectives of the study. These terms are often used interchangeably but we use the term 'aims' to be a broad statement of intention and aspiration and the term 'objectives' to be activity related points along the road to achievement of the aims. The statement of aims should go somewhat further than the statement of the research problem.

Aims
The aims of the example study on attitudes to student status might be the following.

1. To describe attitudes of registered nurses in one hospital to student status for learners.

2. To test a number of hypotheses arising out of attitudes to the proposed move to student status for learners including:
   (a) that age affects attitudes to student status;
   (b) that seniority affects attitudes to student status;
   (c) that graduate nurses have different attitudes to student status than non-graduate nurses; and
   (d) that fears about shortages of trained staff are the major obstacle to approval of the move.

Objectives

1. To review published material relevant to the debate on student status.
2. To select a sample of registered nurses and carry out a postal survey to collect information relevant to the aims of the study.
3. To analyse the data and use it to test the hypotheses described in the aims.
4. To make recommendations about the factors which have been shown through the study to affect attitudes to student status.

Every researcher will formulate aims and objectives slightly differently, but we have no doubt that it is a useful exercise which clarifies for the researcher his or her intentions and purposes in carrying out the study.

Design of the study and choice of methods

You will already have given some thought to design and methods in the earlier stages already described. There is no point in formulating a problem which is too large scale for the available resources, or in setting aims and objectives which you have no hope of achieving. However, it is important to state that as a consequence of this stage of thinking about the detail of design and methods, you may go back and alter your research statement or the aims and objectives. In this sense there is a circularity about the setting up of a research project where every stage depends on previous stages and affects future stages, and you are constantly reassessing the plan as you progress.

Postal survey

A provisional decision has already been made to use a postal survey (which appears in your objectives). You might now give this further consideration. Can you obtain access to a sampling frame (i.e. a list of the total population from which the sample will be drawn), and how big a sample should you have? At this stage it is worth making an initial approach to a senior nursing officer to ask about access. She or he may be unable or unwilling to give you access, in which case your postal survey is a non-starter and you should rethink the methods. Or she or he may feel that to provide you with a sampling frame permission must be obtained from the Health Authority and/or from a hospital committee. The relevant committees may not meet for another three months, which is beyond the time within which the study has to be done. So for a different reason, the postal survey may be an unavailable option. At this point some other approach may be considered.

If access is granted, you need to think about sample size. The technique in Chapter 6 can be used to calculate an appropriate sample size. Suppose that this turns out to be a sample of size 300. The cost of stamps alone will be in the region of £150, taking account of pre-paid return envelopes and follow-up postings. Unless you plan to apply for external funding, this sum may well be outside your means, so the postal survey will have to be dropped on these grounds. What are the alternatives? To interview 300 people face to face would take about 150 hours. You only have two weeks and yourself to carry out interviews. So unless you can recruit a voluntary helper, you may have to drop the interview method altogether. Further, any kind of sampling may be unfeasible. It is worth making the point that sampling is almost always a time consuming process and often a relatively expensive method of doing research. So you may have to use a survey, but not on a random sample. A quota or convenience sample may be used but there are limitations of these approaches in terms of statistical inference. Remember also, when deciding on the number of subjects whether randomly sampled or otherwise that you will have to analyse all this information within the time available.

Clinical trial

If the research design involves a clinical trial, you will be considering different issues at the design stage. A clinical trial is a study of an intervention or treatment involving a patient. Will you be allowed to do it, and whose approval do you need? Again, it is worth making some preliminary contacts at this stage before investing more time in developing the project. Clearance from nursing line management will certainly be needed, but the point at which clearance is granted will vary from one place to another. It must be stressed that we are not here describing the stage of formal communication about a project (which comes later) but are rather suggesting that some 'sounding-out' contacts be made to establish whether it is feasible to proceed with the project at all. It is unlikely that complete clearance to proceed will be given at this point, but you may be told that the project cannot go ahead at all, and it is better to know this sooner rather than later. With any luck you will be told that the project is acceptable in principle, and that full approval to proceed will be considered when you produce more detail of your intentions. For clinical trials or any clinical research involving a patient, you will almost certainly need the co-operation of and/or clearance by the medical profession, and ethical approval must be obtained (see page 25). It may be valuable to take 'soundings' of opinions from these various parties at the design stage of a project. Even if the soundings are not encouraging they may help in re-defining the project in a more acceptable way.

For clinical research you will also need to decide the method of allocation of patients if you are using control and experimental groups. Criteria will have to be identified for the selection of patients for inclusion in the study. Perhaps you will decide, on reflection, that a crossover design can be used (see Chapter 3). These are the kinds of issues to be resolved at the design stage of a clinical project.

Observation

You may on the other hand be planning to observe some aspect of nursing practice – the activity of nurses or patients or both. Such observation where you are a participant is called participant observation, in contrast to non-participant observation where you observe standing outside of the activity. Whichever kind of observation is used you need to think at the design stage about what information is to be collected and recorded. The detail of this of course is the business of the next stage in the research process, the construction of instruments, but it is advisable at the design stage to begin to decide on the types of information to be recorded, and how.

Outcome measures

Consideration of measures of outcome are particularly important. Your research area might be communication between learners and staff nurses. Are you going simply to describe what you observe, or are you going to look at the effectiveness of communication which would involve looking at the outcome of communication. What would the observable results be? One might be implementation of the instructions communicated. Another might be eliciting and comparing the impressions of the two parties to the communication after it had ended. These are questions which should be addressed in principle at the design stage. The detail of exactly how you frame questions and design sheets for recording data can be left to the next stage.

When the design and choice of methods is completed, it is often a useful exercise to try and draw a diagram of your study design. This may reveal gaps or flaws in logic. For example:

Study design – examples

Communication between students and staff nurses
All staff nurses and students on one ward (case study).

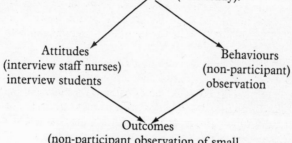

Attitudes
(interview staff nurses)
interview students

Behaviours
(non-participant)
observation

Outcomes
(non-participant observation of small
number of defined outcomes)

Clinical trial on new method of nursing pressure sores

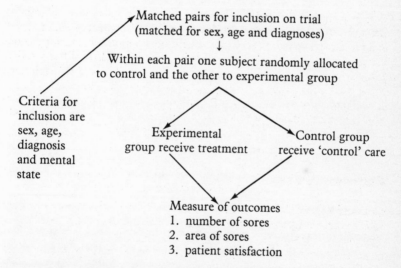

Matched pairs for inclusion on trial
(matched for sex, age and diagnoses)

Within each pair one subject randomly allocated
to control and the other to experimental group

Criteria for
inclusion are
sex, age,
diagnosis
and mental
state

Experimental
group receive treatment

Control group
receive 'control' care

Measure of outcomes
1. number of sores
2. area of sores
3. patient satisfaction

Simple diagrams of this kind will help you to summarise clearly how you
will design the study.

Plans for analysis

In designing a study it is important that you think ahead to your plans for the
analysis. There is no point in producing a complex study design if time or
resources will only enable analysis of part of the data. When the research
design is completed you should be able to state in broad terms the methods of

analysis you will use. Some examples are given below and all statistical tests referred to in this chapter are fully described in later chapters.

Attitudes of registered nurses to student status for learners
Analysis:

1. Description of survey results on main attitudes.
2. Use of χ^2 tests (chi-squared) to examine the relationship between:
   age and attitudes,
   seniority and attitudes,
   graduate status and attitudes,
   reason for attitude and attitudes.

If you plan to use a χ^2 test, remember that there are rules about the size of expected values in cells. Are your numbers going to be big enough to use the χ^2? If your judgment is that the numbers will be too small, you must reconsider either the size of the study or the method of analysis. In this way thinking forward to the analysis may affect your design or even your aims and objectives.

Communication between students and staff nurses
Analysis:

1. Description of attitudes from interview.
2. Description of behaviours from observational data.
3. Description of outcomes from observational data.
4. Identification of behaviours associated with positive outcomes.
5. Identification of behaviours associated with negative outcomes.
6. Test of the hypothesis that the mean number of positive outcomes differs for male and female staff nurses (Mann–Whitney U test, see page 88).

This proposed analysis may suggest to you that further thought is needed to achieve 4 and 5 and this may lead you to reconsider the method by which you record observation of behaviours.

Experimental study of new method of nursing pressure sores
Analysis: test of the hypothesis that at the end of the trial there is no difference between the control and experimental group in

1. number of sores,
2. area of sores,
3. patient satisfaction,

using the Wilcoxon paired signed-ranks test (see page 86).
   The problem with this analysis may be that on reflection you are not confident that you can develop a means of measuring patient satisfaction on an ordinal scale, which is required for a Wilcoxon test (see page 86). You may instead decide to use an nominal scale and use a McNemar test (see page 85). So consideration of the statistical analysis may lead to a change in design.

At this stage of the planning, we would strongly recommend that a statistician is consulted about the proposed design and method of analysis. If you get this wrong and only discover the problem at the analysis stage, the average statistician will not be inclined or may not be able to be helpful! Statisticians like to be consulted at the design stage, because of the implications design has for which statistical method will be possible at the analysis stage.

The importance of the design stage of a study cannot be overstressed in that it is the foundation on which the study is built and it should stimulate every succeeding stage of the study and may well lead to reconsideration of earlier stages.

Funding

You are now at the stage where you can apply for external funding, if necessary. The process of applying for, and being granted, external funding rarely takes less than three months and may take considerably longer, so it may not be feasible at all to make such applications for small scale studies. For these studies you may be able to obtain small amounts of finance from your own hospital, Health Authority or school or college of nursing. However, it must be said that in the present economic climate there is not a lot of spare cash for research available to such bodies.

External funding is awarded by a variety of research councils and charitable trusts. Lists of these can be obtained in libraries. The lists will normally indicate the terms of reference of the awarding body and the scale of funding which is available. Large scale government research councils such as the Medical Research Council or the Economic and Social Research Council have standard and very complex application forms for funding. Most charitable trusts will also have their own application forms which are available on request. However, in some instances you present the submission in your own way.

You need to provide a statement of the research project, its aims and objectives, the design of the study and proposed method of analysis. All of this you will have worked out in the first stages of the research process. In addition the expected outcomes of your project must be explicitly stated – the questions you will be able to answer, and the expected usefulness and relevance of the project.

You should provide two additional sections, one on the timetable and one on the funding you need. An example of a timetable might be:

1st–4th month	construction of questionnaire
5th month	pilot study
6–8th month	data collection
9–14th month	analysis of data
15–18th month	writing of report

If your involvement will be on a part-time basis, you should indicate both the extent of your contribution (e.g. half-time) and the total time period over which the study will extend.

In requesting funding from any body, you will be required to produce an itemised set of estimates. This will obviously depend on the individual study, but in general it is as well to take account of the following possible categories of expenditure:

> salaries (yourself, research assistants),
> travel (to set up project, meet other researchers, collect data),
> typing/clerical support (preparation of instruments and reports),
> photocopying (study instruments),
> equipment (clip boards, test-tubes, white coats etc.),
> costs of analysis (laboratory costs, computing costs),
> postage (particularly for postal survey),
> telephones.

It is obviously helpful if you keep costs to a minimum. Your hospital or college may for example be supportive of your research but unable to give you finance; they may, however, be willing to lend you equipment or let you have free use of clerical resources or of telephones. If you can make clear to an external body that you already have this kind of support it is likely to increase the chance of receiving extra funding from them.

Most funding bodies will consider applications for funding in advance of study instruments being prepared. So you need to describe broadly the content of the proposed questionnaire but not to produce it in finished or even draft form. Some funding bodies – for example the Medical Research Council – insist on ethical approval having already been obtained before funding is awarded. So although we are considering ethical approval as a subsequent stage in the research process it will on occasion need to be carried out before seeking external funding.

If you decide to apply for external funding we strongly advise you to consult a professional researcher for advice on the presentation of your submission. An accountant or finance officer could also be very helpful in advising you on your costings.

Ethical considerations

The area of research ethics is both complex and controversial. There is no generally agreed exhaustive framework for research ethics although there are areas within this on which most researchers would agree. The consideration of research ethics is complicated by the confounding involvement of professional ethics – and ethics are not necessarily standard from one profession to another.

The world was sensitised to the problem of ethics by the infamous so-called medical experiments carried out by Nazi physicians in concentration camps in World War II. More recently there has been considerable public concern about the ethical implications of the thalidomide tragedy and other similar tragedies resulting from use of new drugs.

Research ethics in our field of concern are very much tied up in practice with medical ethics. There are numerous local ethical committees in the UK which have the role of vetting research on ethical grounds. Many of these are in effect medical ethical committees with a majority of the members medically qualified.

It is our view that a great deal more consideration needs to be given to research ethics and that ethical committees should ideally be composed of representatives of a range of health professions, researchers and lay members.

Our concern here, however, is with practicalities. It may be that the nature of your project is such that you need ethical approval (any study involving patients would be an obvious example) or that to obtain co-operation and clearance for your project you have been asked to obtain ethical approval. There is no universally agreed code on when ethical approval should be sought, but many would say that any research involving a patient requires ethical approval. Others would say that only when invasive procedures are involved should such approval be required. This raises the question of what 'invasive' means. Clearly, taking a blood sample is invasive, but what about asking a question in a survey? We can only suggest that you should abide by local guidelines and practices – and these will vary from one locality to another. Seek advice of those in local positions of authority and take the advice given.

If you proceed to apply for ethical approval, you should find out about the procedures from the Chairman or Secretary of your local ethical committee. There will probably be a standard application form.

We would stress, however, that research ethics are not confined to the seeking of approval from ethical committees. Every researcher should be aware of a code of ethics in carrying out research involving patients or the public. In particular the following questionable practices should be avoided (Cook, 1976).

1. Involving people in research without their knowledge or consent.
2. Coercing people to participate.
3. Withholding from the participant the true nature of the research.
4. Leading the research participants to commit acts which diminish their self-respect.
5. Violating the right to self-determination.
6. Exposing the participant to physical or mental stress.
7. Invading the privacy of the participant.
8. Withholding benefits from participants in control groups.
9. Failing to treat participants fairly and to show them consideration and respect.

All of these behaviours raise ethical questions. It is stressed, however, that in some circumstances the potential benefits of research outweigh the costs of questionable practices. But this would have to be justified by the researcher, who should be questioned stringently by the ethical committee.

The principle of 'informed consent' is applied in recruiting subjects into a research study. Senior staff may have agreed that the study can be carried out, but permission must be obtained from the individual participants. The purpose and procedures of the study should be clearly explained and any questions answered before asking permission to include someone. When asking patients, staff or anyone else to participate, it should be made very clear that this is entirely voluntary and refusal to participate will in no way prejudice the care provided to the patient or the standing of the nurse.

A final point on ethics relates to confidentiality. In almost all circumstances people are likelier to co-operate with the researcher if the information is treated in confidence and they can not be identified by name. In virtually all circumstances, the researcher should be able to provide such guarantees. If you can offer such assurance, you should do so, but remember that this places a heavy responsibility on you for the security of data. You must be able to deliver confidentiality if you promise it.

Communications

Well in advance of data collection you will need to obtain formal permission to carry out the study. At an earlier stage some preliminary soundings on the acceptability of the study may have been made but now formal permission to proceed is needed. You should not attempt to obtain permission until you have your own ideas fairly clear. Senior nurse managers, for example, are busy people who want a clear, short and concise statement of what it is you are requesting.

If you want to do nursing research in health service premises we would recommend that you write to the senior nurse in your health authority, and ask with whom you should discuss the project in more detail. You may be referred to a nurse administrator in the authority with special responsibility for research. Once this person has approved the project write to the senior nurse at district, hospital and unit level for every hospital, educational or community setting you wish to include in the study. A standard letter will suffice which explains the project and asks if you may now approach individual staff for interviews or to discuss with them your plans for data collection.

If you are planning to observe activity, staff or patients, it is well worth meeting with the nursing staff in advance and gaining their co-operation and acceptance. You should expect some reservations on their part – few people would initially feel comfortable with the notion that a researcher is watching and recording information about their professional practice. Answer questions directly and honestly and try to get to know staff personally. A brief information sheet about the project available should be given to nursing staff and other interested parties.

Formal medical clearance will be needed if the study impinges on medical care or involves patients. If so, the same communication process should be used, making the initial approach to the senior medical officer at Regional level and working downwards. In our experience it is best not to depend on information about your study being passed 'down the line'. It is safer to communicate directly with each tier yourself.

You may need ethical clearance for certain kinds of studies as described earlier.

Closer to the time of data collection, but allowing reasonable consultation time, you should write to the trade unions and to doctors (if they have not yet been involved) at ward level. In each case a brief and courteous letter for information is appropriate. You can offer to provide more detail if requested. Remember the particular interest of each party. Unions will be concerned that your study will not damage the working conditions of their members; doctors will be concerned that the research does not include assessment of medical practice or unauthorised access to medical notes. They will also want to ensure the well-being of patients – as indeed will the nursing staff. The nursing staff will want to know what you intend to do and they will be concerned about confidentiality since they are the main focus of many nursing research studies.

It is also a good idea to prepare a short information sheet for the patients involved if you are researching in a ward, or indeed in the community.

While all of this may seem somewhat cumbersome, its importance cannot be overemphasised. If you skimp on communication you will probably be in the centre of a row in a short time. If properly informed, people are normally helpful and co-operative.

Construction of instruments

You are now ready to begin sampling, or identifying patients for your clinical trial, but concurrently you should be working on your research instruments. This term covers everything from questionnaires to forms for recording observations. It is worth going back to published papers at this point and looking at other researchers' instruments, which are often included as appendices. It may be possible to use whole schedules or parts of schedules and provided you seek permission and acknowledge the original researcher this is perfectly acceptable, in fact desirable.

If new instruments have to be developed, some of the techniques in the next chapter should be useful. The design of questionnaires is discussed there. The use of the Delphi method is recommended if you want to develop an instrument for assessing clinical practice or outcomes.

In developing any instrument it is helpful to imagine yourself in the situation where the instrument will be used. Will your results fit into the format you are prescribing? Have you left enough space to record the likely answer to a question or the event under observation?

Also very important in construction of instruments is consideration of the analysis. Does the form lend itself to easy collation and analysis? Do you need a column of space on the right to add up scores? For questionnaires in particular you should have space on the right (about 1 inch wide) for coding boxes if your results are going onto a computer or for clerical work if not. Head this space 'For office use only' at the top of each page of a questionnaire.

Having produced a draft of the instrument it may be helpful to do a mini-pilot study. If it is a questionnaire try it out on friends or colleagues. If it is a form for recording observations, try it out yourself in a ward, or ask a nurse colleague to try it out for you. In this way you can probably improve your instrument. It normally takes several drafts of an instrument before you yourself will feel happy with it.

Pilot study

Having cleared the way by communicating in advance with all parties, you can carry out a pilot study. The purpose of this is to try out the study instruments and to test out the feasibility of the data collection process. The pilot study should be carried out on a small group of subjects or in a small area outside that included in your main study. Examining the results of the pilot study will identify problems in the wording of questions or the recording of data and will help you to improve the study instruments. Ideally, if the instruments are altered you should carry out a second pilot study, but time and resources often preclude this.

In this same period, training of any helpers to be involved in the data collection should be carried out. You may find it helpful to draw up instructions or guidelines for the helpers to help to ensure that everyone is operating on the same basis.

Data collection

If you have got everything right up to this point, everything should go smoothly! Data collection is surprisingly hard work. If you spend all day interviewing people, you will feel very tired at the effort of being bright and warm and encouraging to every respondent. Ward observation can also be very tiring since you must concentrate constantly lest you miss any part of the picture. The easiest types of study from the data collection viewpoint are the postal survey and the experimental clinical study. These demand least human contact on the part of the researcher.

When carrying out non-participant observation on a ward, as a trained nurse, you may be faced by occasional dilemmas when patients ask you for some service, or have some need which you perceive. In these circumstances we recommend that you refer the request to a member of the nursing staff – if necessary relay the request yourself. In exceptional circumstances where a patient is in immediate danger and you are the only person in the vicinity you must, as a trained nurse, intervene. It may, however, subsequently be necessary to withdraw as a researcher – either because your intervention is resented or not understood, or because by becoming involved yourself you have altered the pattern of activity under study.

It will pay dividends if you can find time to organise your data as it is collected. It is very daunting at the end of a period of data collection to find that you have amassed hundreds of sheets of paper. Each sheet should of course have identifying information on it – ward, or health centre, date, name of observer or interviewer – but even so, it is a good idea to file it in some ordered fashion as it is collected.

Analysis

This will depend on the methods chosen and methods of analysis which should have been largely determined at the design stage. However, once you start to analyse data unexpected and interesting findings will generate extra analysis.

If you intend to analyse results with no more technology than a pocket calculator, you will find it helpful to transfer the data onto master sheets. For example, all the responses to each question in a survey should be placed on one sheet. Then it is relatively easy to calculate frequency distributions and summary statistics. If you have access to a computer, all of that can be done once you have the data in the system. In this case the initial tasks will be coding the results into a form acceptable to the computer and having the coded data punched onto computer filestore tape, or yourself punching in data at a terminal, followed by learning how to analyse the data.

We would strongly recommend that however you analyse results, you date each sheet of paper and also keep notes on your thinking. It is very easy to cover sheet after sheet of paper and then to go back after a break and find your own meanderings incomprehensible! This is especially true of big scale projects where the analysis takes months or even years.

Presentation of findings

This can take a variety of forms and one project may well be presented in a variety of ways for different audiences. Normally there is one initial report to be written – perhaps for the course you are taking, or for the body which funded the work or for the staff who co-operated in the work. You must decide on the priority.

Irrespective of the reader or readers to whom the report is directed, the content should follow the research process as described in this chapter. You need to state the research problem, provide a literature review and state the aims and objectives of the study and describe the research design. A brief account of communications is usually of interest and you should acknowledge any funding you received. If ethical approval was acquired, this can be briefly reported.

Rather than describing research instruments in detail you can append them. The pilot study warrants a brief description, as does the data collection. But the main interest of the report is the analysis and findings and most of the report should probably be devoted to these. However, if this is a research report being submitted for a degree then more detail on the research methods will be needed.

Most reports conclude with a discussion of the findings and a consideration of the implications of the research for policy or practice. A list of references should be provided at the end.

If you hope to publish the work in an academic journal it is worth looking at other published papers for style and presentation. Most journals have guidelines about layout and length and there are standard ways of citing references.

The use of appropriate language in a report is very important. If writing for nurses you will not need to explain what the 'nursing process' is, but you certainly will need to if you publish in an applied statistical journal! In general keep language as simple as possible. Over elaborate use of language is often perceived as – and often is – a smokescreen for sloppiness in the research itself.

Having produced reports to meet your immediate obligations we would urge you to provide a short account of your findings for those who have co-operated in the study – perhaps the staff of the ward or health centre. This will be greatly appreciated and it will smooth the path of the next researcher who approaches this area. People do not like to feel that they are just the fodder for researchers. The major reason for disseminating your results is the hope that your work will help others in achieving higher professional standards.

Summary

This chapter covered the various stages of the research process. In trying to cover all situations, we may have made the process seem more lengthy than it usually is. Some of the stages may well not be relevant to some projects.

We hope that we have not discouraged any would-be nursing researchers from taking the plunge, for our intention is the opposite. We believe that this logical approach to tackling a problem can be applied by any practising nurse in her own working situation. The approach is as valid in addressing small local problems as it is in investigating major issues. The examples given have tended to be relatively complex to enable illustration of potential problems, but many practical problems are simple to define and research. The important thing is to use the logic of the research process, and let facts speak for themselves.

The Briggs Report (1972) recommended that nursing should be a research based profession. It did not imply that every nurse should be a professional researcher. But an understanding of the research process and the confidence and commitment to translate it into valuable and practical everyday use will bring the nursing profession some considerable way towards meeting Briggs' aspiration.

3

Research Techniques

Introduction

For someone starting out to do research, one of the great dilemmas is how to choose the appropriate research technique from the 57 varieties which seem to be available. In fact the inexperienced researcher often focuses initially on the technique at the expense of the research problem itself. The desired order of events, described in some detail in the previous chapter, is first to define the problem, its aims and objectives; then the selection of the research technique should follow relatively easily.

In this chapter nursing research techniques are placed within a wider framework; three kinds of nursing research are identified and some techniques associated with each are explored in more detail.

One of the reasons why nursing research methods seem so complex and varied is because nursing research spans such a range of traditional research approaches. Nursing research can be about people – the nursing staff or patients – and this falls within conventional social science methodology. Or nursing research can involve laboratory based measurements, for example, the carrying out of biochemical tests. In this instance, the techniques will be drawn from scientific research. Or nursing research can be a qualitative, in-depth case-study in one ward or community location, in which case it falls within the ethnographic tradition associated with the humanities. In some instances the evaluation of new methods of management of patient problems are evaluated in ways comparable to those used in medical research, i.e. clinical trials.

Research spectrum

Nursing research can therefore be placed along any point of the spectrum of traditional research methods:

Scientific research (controlled laboratory experiments)	Medical research (clinical trials)	Social science (people, surveys)	Ethnographic research (case studies)

Research in the scientific mould tends to be undertaken in laboratory conditions entirely controlled by the researcher. Clinical trials normally take place in the real world with real patients, but conditions are partially controlled by the research. The social science researcher tries most often to carry out research on the world as it is, so the conditions are mostly outside the control of the researcher, and the same kind of conditions would pertain in ethnographic research.

It follows that the skills required of the researcher are rather different as we move across the research spectrum. Increasing social and communication skills are needed as we move from left to right, and there is also an increase in the degree of subjective judgement required at the right hand end of the spectrum. These are factors which should be borne in mind when choosing research techniques – because, although a particular research problem will often fall clearly into one of the four categories described, there will also not uncommonly be room for choice of technique, particularly between the social science survey based approach and the ethnographic approach. In addition, many problems are very complex and require the use of more than one technique.

This taxonomy of research approaches provides a framework within which more detailed attention will be given to the various kinds of nursing research. It is suggested that most published nursing research could be classified in at least one of the following ways:

1. *Attitude/opinion survey* – these focus on what nurses or patients think or feel about particular topics or issues and frequently involve the use of questionnaires. Factual and personal/social information will often also be collected. For example, a survey of patient satisfaction with care might cover personal, clinical and social information about the patient as well as the patient's attitudes about the care received.
2. *Clinical practice and evaluation* – these studies are concerned with what nurses do, and how effectively they do it. Included in this category would be clinical trials of new methods of management of patient problems, observation of nurses and nursing practice, studies of work through diaries or by researchers, epidemiological and community health studies and laboratory based scientific studies involving laboratory measurement of clinical parameters influenced by nursing activities.
3. *The organisation of nursing* – these studies focus on organisational issues and would include studies of manpower, studies of systems of working,

allocation of nurses, allocation of resources, cost-effectiveness and cost-benefit studies, and studies of the training system.

It should be stressed that many studies will fall into more than one of the above categories. For example, a study of nurse training in Northern Ireland (Reid, 1986) surveyed staff and student attitudes (1 above), used schedules to assess learner performance and studied work patterns (2 above) and assessed manpower and other resources available to wards (3 above). The three categories are useful, however, in identifying ranges of related research techniques. The following sections deal with each area in turn, selecting the most commonly used or potentially useful research techniques for more detailed discussion.

Attitude/opinion surveys

A survey normally involves the use of questionnaires as the research instrument. The same questions in the same format are asked of every respondent. The respondents are often asked to provide responses in a predetermined form – by ticking from lists of possible responses – but some questions can also be answered in free form in any way the respondent wishes.

Surveys are most often carried out on samples of people from wider populations. But there is no reason why a survey should necessarily be carried out on a sample. If your resources and time allow it, you can survey an entire population, or you could use the same type of questionnaire with a very small number of people in a case study. In most instances, however, samples are selected for surveys, so we will first describe some of the most commonly used methods of sampling.

Sampling

Having defined your research problem, you must then define the population for your study. For example, if you want to study nurse training for the register in Northern Ireland, your population might be all students in training in Northern Ireland on 1st January, 1987. If you want to study training for the roll in the UK, your population would be all pupils in training in the UK on 1st January, 1987. (Note that although the dates in these examples are arbitrarily chosen the date does affect the population, so it should be part of the definition.) If you want to study staffing levels in a particular hospital, your population might be all wards in the hospital.

Having identified and defined the population, the next step is to obtain access to a *sampling frame*. This is a list of every member of your population. For the examples of populations just given, the respective sampling frames would be a list of all Northern Ireland students in training (probably requested from the National Board for Nursing, Midwifery and Health

Visiting or from the Colleges of Nursing), a list of all UK pupils in training (from the equivalent UK bodies), and a list of all the wards in the hospital.

Simple random sampling

The simplest form of sampling is called simple random sampling. This method ensures that every member of the sampling frame has an equal chance of selection. This form of sampling can be done in at least three ways.

1. By writing the name of each member of the population on a small card and drawing cards out of a hat. This obviously becomes time-consuming with large populations.
2. By using random number tables – Neave (1981), for example, contains a set of random numbers. If you number the members of your sampling frame, the tables will then tell you which numbers to select.
3. By using a number of easily available computer programs to produce random numbers and proceed as 2.

The question now arises – how big should your sample be? This is the question most often asked of statisticians by those new to social survey based research. It is possible to estimate sample size mathematically. This is done by first stating what is expected of the sample in terms of desired limits of error. This is a judgement which must be made by the researcher. On drug trials, for example, because the cost of error could be human suffering or even death, a much smaller margin of error would be acceptable than in an opinion survey. Once the acceptable level of error is stated, the appropriate sample size can be estimated. We will illustrate how this can be done with a simple example. A researcher wishes to look at the requirements for blood transfusion supplies in a hospital. She surveys a simple random sample of patients. The most important question relates to the blood group. She needs to know the proportion of patients with blood group 'O'. She states that this proportion in the sample would need to be within 5% of the proportion in the population, that is if the proportion for all patients in the population is 50%, the sample proportion must be within the range 45–55%. She must also make a guess (as informed as possible) about the proportion in the population. For example, she may know from other studies that this is likely to lie between 30% and 60%. The estimated sample size, n, is then given by

$$n = \frac{4PQ}{E^2}$$

where P is the estimate of the percentage of people with blood group 'O' in the whole population (i.e. in the hospital),

$Q = 1 - P$
E = margin of error acceptable in either direction.

So, if P is 30, Q is 70 and PQ is 2100, and if P is 60, Q is 40 and PQ is 2400.

The value of P in the 30–60% range which gives the biggest value of PQ is P = 50%, Q = 50%. To be on the safe side, take PQ = 2500. So,

$$n = \frac{4 \times 2500}{25} = 400$$

and a sample of size 400 should be drawn.

Applying this method to the key variable in a sample survey should produce a desirable sample size. It may be of course that your resources and time will not allow you to cover a sample of this size, so you may have to trade accuracy for savings in money or time. Simple random sampling should provide you with sample means which are good estimates of population means, and sample proportions which are good estimates of population proportions.

Stratified random sampling
Another common method of sampling is stratified random sampling (SRS). This is appropriate when the population contains subpopulations – for example, the list of all Northern Ireland general student nurses would contain six subpopulations, one for each College of Nursing which offers general training. The intention of SRS is to sample independently from each subpopulation. So rather than taking say, a 10% sample from all Northern Ireland students irrespective of college, you could sample 10% from each college, thus ensuring that each college was equitably represented in terms of its size. To carry out SRS, you obviously must be able to divide your sampling frame into the appropriate subpopulations before sampling. Note that you do not have to take the same percentage sample from every subpopulation. You might wish to sample twice as many proportionately from one college as from another. In this case, however, you should consult a textbook of sampling (e.g. Cochrane, 1977) to check how to calculate means and other sample statistics.

Stratified random sampling is sometimes chosen for reasons of practical convenience – for example, different types of sampling frames may exist in the subpopulations – but also because in heterogeneous populations, it is a way to improve estimates of population parameters by setting up strata, each of which is internally relatively homogeneous.

Cluster sampling
A third widely used method of sampling is cluster sampling. This is when clusters containing smaller units are selected, rather than direct selection of the smaller units. For example, if we want to survey attitudes to the service provided by general practitioners in Scotland, it might be decided to have a sample size of 5000. Five thousand people randomly selected from the whole of Scotland will provide a very scattered sample, with subjects hundreds of miles apart. The costs of fieldwork would be prohibitive. Instead, GP lists could be considered as clusters and five of these randomly

selected from all GP lists in Scotland. Depending on list size, every person or a random sample of persons on those five lists would be included to give about 5000 total subjects. Cluster sampling is often used for practical and logistical benefits such as described in this example.

The three methods of sampling described thus far all use *probability sampling*. By this we mean that we know the probability of inclusion of each subject in the study. The level of precision of the summary statistics provided from the sample can then be calculated. The final methods of sampling mentioned here do not have this advantage. Quota sampling is, however, widely used in market research and in opinion polls.

Quota sampling

Quota sampling requires the researchers to state how many subjects with defined characteristics are required. For example, 20 men aged 50–60 in social class two, or 20 women aged 20–30 in social class four. The person collecting the survey data then has to find any 20 people in her geographical patch with the required characteristics. In other words, selection of subjects within a defined group is not random. They are quite likely, for example, to be people personally known to the person collecting the information! The problem with this method lies in the lack of randomness, and the inability to calculate the precision of sample summary statistics. The quota method can produce samples which are biased on characteristics like income, education and occupation.

Convenience sampling

Convenience sampling also provides no probabilistic or inferential potential. In this case, the sample comprises subjects who are simply available in a convenient way to the researcher. There is no randomness, and the likelihood of bias is quite high. Results cannot be generalised to any wider population. However, this method is often the only feasible one, particularly for students or others with restricted time and resources, and can be legitimately used, provided its limitations are clearly understood and stated.

It is highly desirable when sampling to understand the broad principles of the method you use. In practice, it is often necessary to compromise on the selection of your sample, but the important thing is to state this clearly, understand the limitations that are placed on your findings and do not make extravagant claims for the results. It may be worth restating the enormous benefit of carrying out a survey of a random sample of 20 people as opposed to surveying 20 people who are not a sample. In the former case, you can generalise your results to the entire population from which your 20 subjects were selected, so you may be able to speak with authority about hundreds of people. In the latter case, you only have information on twenty people who may not be representative of any wider group at all.

Questionnaire design

Method of administration

Having decided on the method of sampling (if indeed sampling is to be used) the other main technique in the area of attitude/opinion surveys is that of questionnaire design. The first question to consider is how you intend to administer the questionnaire. The cheapest method is generally the postal survey. The main costs are in the time taken to fill envelopes and dispatch them and the costs of postage. Face-to-face surveys can be very expensive since you will probably have to pay for the time and travel of fieldwork assistants. The main disadvantage of the postal questionnaire is that response rates tend to be low, and significantly lower than those from face-to-face surveys. It is easier not to post back a survey form than to refuse to co-operate with a personal interviewer who has asked for your help!

The problem with low response rates, whether on postal or face-to-face surveys is that there may be bias in the responses you do receive: those who reply may be different in some key respect from those who do not. If your response rate is low – say 50% or less – it is useful if you can compare your responders and non-responders on one or two key variables. You may, for example, be able to check the age and grade of non-responders from some other source, and compare these to the age and grade distribution of your responders. If the distributions look similar on one or two key variables, this is supporting evidence (although not proof) that your sample is not biased.

In choosing a postal or face-to-face method, another key question relates to the type of material your survey will include. If, for example, subjects will be helped to respond by consulting other people, the mail survey is preferable. The same holds if a considered rather than an immediate response is required. Some people will answer personal or sensitive questions more readily when not face-to-face with an interviewer who is a stranger. Mail surveys also avoid the problem of the effects of different interviewers, since often face-to-face interviews require several interviewers to cover a sample. The impact of individual interviewers then becomes a problem.

The mail survey also has limitations. It can only be used with simple and straightforward questions which are likely to be totally comprehensible to the sample being studied. It could not be used, for example, in a study which might include illiterate or senile or mentally handicapped people, or children. The answers provided in a postal survey are final – there is no opportunity to probe further or check that questions have been understood. You can never be certain exactly who has completed a mail questionnaire. There are further limitations like the lack of opportunity to observe extra relevant factors and record them, but the most serious limitation of the postal survey is probably the tendency to produce low response rates.

Apart from doing some checks on the non-responders little can be done after the event. However, there are a number of ways to increase the response rate from postal surveys. The use of one, or even better, two follow-up postings to the non-responders will normally provide a substantial increase in response rate. To do this, you must be able to identify respondents' returns. If you use codes on the questionnaires, you will need a master list of codes attached to names, so that you can tick off responders as you receive their returns.

Sponsorship of a survey by some body which the respondent is likely to respect has been shown to increase response rates. For example, sponsorship by DHSS or by a National Board might well increase responses from a postal survey of nurses. Sometimes a payment or gift can be offered as an incentive to response, and this is likely to increase response rates. Finally, keep the postal survey as short as possible. The shorter it is the better the response rate is likely to be.

The face-to-face interview provides better response rates. The training of the interviewer in making the initial approach to the subject is very important. Nowadays it can be useful to expose interviewers to social skills training using close circuit television as an aid to identification of problems in communication. The direct contact between interviewer and subject has an immense benefit in allowing the interviewer to probe for more informa-tion or to elaborate on a question. The interviewer is also free to record any relevant or interesting information outside the immediate range of questions in the questionnaire. In fact some information can be recorded without asking any questions at all, for instance sex of the respondent. There are fewer constraints on the length of the interview – some face-to-face interviews take up to an hour although about 30 minutes would in general seem to be a reasonable length to aim for.

We have then two main methods, the postal and face-to-face method. It may be worth mentioning that a third method, interviews by telephone, is now being widely used in the USA. This has led to problems, however, because not all of the populations under study have telephones, so studies are necessarily biased towards more affluent households. The telephone method would not be suitable for a population sample survey in the UK for the same reasons, but it could possibly be used to interview a professional group at work. We do not recommend it for surveys of nurses, however, as we cannot imagine the average very busy nurse taking kindly to a request for a 15 minute phone interview during working hours!

Some practical points

When carrying out a postal survey:

1. Always include pre-paid return envelopes with each questionnaire.
2. If you are using codes instead of names, code the questionnaires before they go out and keep a masterlist of codes and names if you want to send follow-up questionnaires to non-responders.
3. Always include a covering letter, explaining why you are doing the survey.

When carrying out a face-to-face survey:

1. Make sure that if more than one person is carrying out the interviews, they are trained to do so in the same way.

2. If possible, contact subjects in advance to let them know when you would like to interview them.
3. If people refuse, be as persuasive as you can, but in the end you must respect their right not to participate, and withdraw courteously.

Questionnaire content

We now come to the content of the questionnaires. It is obvious that content and style will depend on whether the survey is postal or face-to-face. In the latter case, for example, you do not need to ask a person for their sex (and would look foolish if you did!). The best guide here is common sense, and a careful pilot study. In general, the postal survey must stand by itself and be totally clear in what it asks and how responses should be made. So instructions are very important – for example, 'tick one of the items' or 'circle the response which best represents your opinion'. In a face-to-face interview, only the interviewer needs to understand the method of recording answers to questions.

The first stage in developing the content of the questionnaire should be to identify the issues which you wish to examine. For example, if you want to survey the attitudes of ward sisters to ward based teaching of learners, the issues to be covered might include:

> the numbers of learners allocated,
> the staffing level of the ward,
> liaison with the college/school of nursing,
> courses attended relevant to teaching,
> age and experience of sister,
> views about the role of learners

You will almost certainly identify more issues than you can reasonably include. The most common mistake is to be tempted to ask about everything. Be disciplined and cut the issues down to the essential. Bear in mind that you will have to analyse all this information!

Having identified the issues, construct some questions to elicit the kind of information you would like on each issue. Again you should probably reduce the total at this stage! Then look at the order in which the questions should be asked.

In our experience people find personal questions on age or employment status or occupation quite threatening. Although it seems intuitively sensible to begin with what to you is background information, you will do better to place these questions last. We would recommend that you begin with some unthreatening factual questions which are clearly relevant to the subject area of your survey. For example, for the study of ward sister attitudes towards learners you could first ask: 'How many students are normally allocated to your ward?' You may well want to establish the sister's level of education later in the interview, but she may well resent the question and might not immediately see the relevance of it to your topic. Such questions are best placed later in the questionnaire.

In general, the order of questions should follow a logical pattern where possible, in such a way that the respondent will be aware of the relationship between topics. If you are interested in specific issues, it can be helpful to start with questions on broader issues and then narrow down to the specific. This is called a funnel sequence of questions. For example, on the issue of liaison between ward sisters and tutors:

> Do you ever visit the school of nursing?
> If yes, how often?
> Who do you see there?

If you are interested in broader issues a reverse funnel sequence can be useful, leading the respondent from the particular to the general:

> Do you like teaching learners?
> Did your training prepare you to be a teacher?

Sometimes a 'no' response to the first of a series of questions will invalidate the remainder of this series which is aimed at positive responders. In this case instruct your interviewer to move on to the next relevant question, or in a postal survey, place clear directions for the respondent, such as 'if "No" please proceed to question 14'.

Questions can be open or closed. An open question allows the respondent to decide freely on the level of detail and content of his answer. Such responses may be tedious and difficult to analyse. There are instances where it is not appropriate to provide predetermined alternative responses for the subject to choose (closed questions) – either because you cannot predict at all what the responses might be, or because you want a full response – but we would recommend that you keep open questions to a minimum. With closed questions you can always leave a blank line for people to record any other response not covered by your set of possible responses.

It is impossible to list or even summarise the plethora of published guidelines on question wording. There are, however, some important basic points to remember.

1. Be as specific as possible.
2. Use simple language.
3. Make sure that you only ask one question in each item.
4. Avoid words like 'and' and 'or' – you may well be asking two questions if one of these words appears.
5. Avoid vague words like 'regularly' or 'frequently' – they mean different things to different people. You should specify frequency or regularity through use of a closed question.
6. Avoid leading questions: 'Do you think that the UKCC is right to opt for student status?' invites a 'yes' answer whereas 'Should the UKCC have risked its standing by opting for student status?' invites the answer 'no'.
7. Avoid presuming questions – the best known example of which is 'When did you stop beating your wife?'.
8. Be careful of questions concerning frequency of behaviour, e.g. 'When did you last visit the school of nursing?', 'How often on average do you

visit the school of nursing?' and 'How often have you visited the school of nursing in the last year?' These are quite different questions. You must decide which it is you want to ask.

Having designed your questionnaire, you should pilot it as described in the previous chapter, first, perhaps on friends or colleagues and secondly on a group similar to, but not including, the study group. The pilot may lead you to reword or re-design the questionnaire.

The intention in this brief outline of questionnaire design has been to provide a readable summary of the technique. For a fuller exposition we refer you to *Survey Methods in Social Investigation* by C. Moser and G. Kalton (1972) on which this section has drawn.

Clinical practice and evaluation

A good deal of published nursing research would fall into this category, but it is a very wide category in terms of the techniques which might be used. Sample surveys, for example, although more closely associated with the previous category of research into attitudes and opinions might well also be used in the evaluation of clinical practice on the part of the nurse or the patient. Surveys could also be used to investigate community health issues or to gather information for epidemiological studies. A good deal of research on clinical practice involves the design of simple pro-formas on which to collect structured information. There are no general guidelines which can be given about the construction of such pro-formas, it is simply a matter of being clear about the information required and designing a suitable form as concisely and neatly as possible.

There are two techniques on which we will provide some detail; one, clinical trials because they are increasingly widely used in clinical research and the other, the Delphi technique, because of its enormous potential value in nursing research.

Clinical trials

It is important that new drugs or treatments are properly and scientifically tested before being made generally available. The standard method of research design is the clinical trial. This has been widely used in medical research, but is increasingly being recognised by nurse researchers as a technique for evaluating advances and innovations in nursing care.

There are normally two groups: the control group and the treatment group. It is essential that these groups are as similar as is possible in all relevant respects. In some cases patients are 'matched' in pairs for age, social class, sex, primary diagnosis and perhaps other factors. One member of each pair is randomly assigned to the treatment group and one to the control group. If matching is not carried out, the patients are randomly allocated to either treatment or control group. The patients in the control group receive either the standard conventional treatment or a placebo if there is no conventional treatment available. Ideally neither patient nor professional practitioner should know which patient is in the treatment group and which is in the control group. In this instance the trial is called a 'double-blind' trial. However, while this may be feasible in drug trials it is difficult to envisage 'double-blind' trials in nursing research. Nevertheless, the use of assistants in collecting data who *are not* aware of which group the patient is in, is feasible and greatly strengthens the research design.

Sometimes the patient can be used as his own control, particularly with a chronic stable condition. The patient is exposed to either treatment or control; then after a time lapse which is long enough for any treatment effects to disappear but short enough to ensure no change in his condition, he is then exposed to the alternative regime. This is called a 'crossover' trial. Half of the patients have the placebo or conventional treatment first, and the remainder the new treatment first.

There will almost always be ethical considerations in this kind of research. Approval from an appropriate ethical body should be obtained.

Having designed the trial, the treatment and placebo regimes are carried out, and predefined outcomes are measured. These might be hours of pain or size of lesion or area of a sore. The analysis is then a straightforward comparison of the results for the two groups. Significance tests of the kind described in Chapter 5 would be appropriate. Non-parametric methods are likely to be suitable both because outcome measures may well not be Normally distributed and because the numbers in clinical trials tend to be small. For clinical trials with matched pairs of subjects the Wilcoxon test might well be suitable, and with matched groups the Mann–Whitney test would be appropriate (see Chapter 5).

Clinical trials are quite simple in terms of design and the logistics of carrying them out. The main difficulty is in matching the experimental with a suitable control group. It is surprisingly difficult to find patients of sufficiently similar characteristics. You can obviously improve your trial by controlling as much as possible, for example using only one ward to avoid the effect of different medical and nursing personnel. The point is, as far as possible, to make standard any factor other than the treatment which might affect the outcome.

It may take quite a while to obtain enough subjects to conduct a clinical trial. Not all patients will be suitable on clinical or other grounds, to enter the trial. Often you need volunteers, and it is possible that not all patients who are suitable will agree to enter the trial.

Nurses could use this approach as a research technique in a variety of ways, in the course of the normal delivery of care. Most nurses have views about new and better ways to care for patients and the clinical trial offers a route to an objective assessment of innovation.

The Delphi method

This is a technique which can be used to incorporate professional judgement into the design of research instruments. The role of professional judgement in research is a topic which has attracted very little attention in the literature, yet it raises fundamental questions. Is it legitimate for a qualified nurse to exercise her professional judgement as part of a research programme or project? We believe that this detracts from the perceived objectivity of the research, however 'correct' the professional judgement might be.

The Delphi method is aimed at obtaining a consensus of professional judgement from a panel of experts. The method arose from the recognition that if any group of people tries to achieve consensus in a face-to-face situation, the consensus reached will be heavily dependent on the interplay of personalities. The Delphi method therefore uses a postal exchange of information from a central co-ordinator to each expert. The panel never meet each other and only communicate with each other through the co-ordinator.

Reid (1986) used this technique to develop schedules to measure learner performance. She wished to assess the performance of learners on a small number of selected procedures at the end of a clinical allocation. Nine procedures were chosen and one of them, the bedbath, will illustrate the method.

The nurse researcher on the team drew up a list of observable behaviours in the execution of a bedbath. Certain criteria were laid down in advance about the type of patient involved. Altogether some eighty items were included to provide what the nurse researcher regarded as a perfect bed-bathing procedure. This is the first stage of the Delphi method – placing a simple structure on the problem.

A team of experts had been identified. These were clinical teachers and tutors in the Province's Colleges of Nursing who had been involved in devising similar schedules for ward based assessments. The draft form which the nurse researcher produced was posted to each expert who was asked to (a) add any desired items, (b) delete any undesirable items, and (c) provide a weight between one and ten for each item indicating its relative importance. In this way items concerning the safety of patients might be given a score close to 10 while items of low importance would be given correspondingly lower scores. The panel were encouraged to discuss the task with their own colleagues but not with other panel members, and then post a response to the researchers.

The consensus of opinion was identified and those items on which there was no consensus were returned to the panel members along with the range of opinion received. Members were asked to consider these points again and post back a further response. This process was repeated until complete consensus had been achieved.

Consensus on nine such test schedules was achieved on three rounds. This supports our belief that the Delphi technique is a very successful means of obtaining professional consensus views from nurses. The resulting research instrument had an objectivity which it could never have claimed had only the nurse researcher been involved. A second important benefit was that because a good number of nurse educators were involved in this way in the design of the instrument it gained considerable credibility in the eyes of the profession.

This technique has enormous potential for a wide range of nursing research problems. To evaluate any aspect of nursing practice, you could draw up a structured assessment and use a Delphi panel to validate it. The members of the panel could be your own colleagues if they are experts in the clinical area of interest. Provided they do not discuss the instrument with each other they can be on the Delphi panel.

The organisation of nursing

Studies of the organisation of nursing may well have less immediate appeal than clinical or survey based research projects, but they are of very considerable immediate value in the age of cost-cutting and resource shrinkage. The advent of the general manager makes it doubly imperative for nurses to be able to defend or increase their resources by putting forward well considered and well presented evidence.

Much of this kind of research can be done using already collected and available information. The next section will be devoted to techniques applied to routine data sources. Sometimes new information needs to be collected, however, so the final section describes a technique which provides a wealth of detailed information on nursing activity and could be applied in a variety of circumstances.

Routinely available information

The off-duty rota

From the off-duty rota you can add up for a day or a week the number of nursing hours provided by each grade of nurse employed in a ward. You can then calculate the ratio of trained staff to learners, the ratio of unqualified to qualified nurses or the proportion of trained staff. This would be a useful exercise over time for one ward because changes in these ratios could easily be identified if they were plotted on graphs. The mix of skills available to a ward can be described in detail from this kind of study.

The bed state form

From this form a number of important indices of workload can be calculated. Some of these are already routinely calculated in medical record offices, but they are rarely relayed back to wards, or used by nurses. Over 30 days, the following information could easily be extracted from the bed state forms.

1. Total number of occupied beds.
2. Total number of available beds (the total bed complement of the ward).
3. Total number of deaths and discharges.

You can now calculate a number of useful indices.

(a) Bed occupancy $= \dfrac{\text{total occupied beds}}{\text{total available beds}} \times 100$

(b) Throughput $= \dfrac{\text{total deaths and discharges}}{\text{average available beds}}$

(c) Average length of stay $= \dfrac{\text{total occupied beds}}{\text{total deaths and discharges}}$

(d) Turnover interval $= \dfrac{\text{total available beds} - \text{total occupied beds}}{\text{total deaths and discharges}}$

If these indices are kept each month for a ward, they provide a valuable record of the work of the ward. If, for example, bed occupancy increases from 70% to 90% and stays at the higher level for some months, a graph showing this trend would be valuable ammunition if it is felt that more staff are required.

The off-duty rota and the bed state form
Using both these sources, you can easily calculate the nursing hours per patient for a day in one ward. This is done by dividing the available nursing hours by the number of occupied beds. If over time you find a lot of fluctuation in this index, it may be advisable to investigate the allocation of staff and make it more even, day by day. Studies of this kind have been carried out in hundreds of wards, and the nurses who work in those wards are always amazed at the inexplicable variations from day to day. This simple technique could ensure that the best possible allocation of staff is achieved.

These are just some examples of the use to which routine locally available information can be put.

Activity analysis

Studies of organisational aspects of nursing will sometimes require purpose collected information on who is doing what, when, with whom and to whom. An excellent but little used technique for such observation is called activity analysis.

Activity analysis is carried out by observing each nurse in turn within a predetermined time cycle. The time cycle is fixed to allow each nurse to be observed briefly, so factors like the structure of the ward and the number of nurses on duty will determine the cycle. In our experience most wards can be covered in cycles lasting between 10 and 30 minutes.

As each nurse is observed a number of aspects of her activity are recorded.

The aspects have been determined in advance and a special form designed on which to record the information. For example you might record
the grade of the nurse under observation,
the grade of any other nurse she is working with,
the nursing activity,
the name of the patient (if any),
whether teaching or learning is occurring.
Nursing activity can be placed in a standard 35-category classification. For a fuller explanation of this technique see Reid (1986).

These observations are carried out on each nurse in turn within every time cycle. This should continue without pause for twelve hours on at least three separate days. At the end, you will have thousands of observations of nursing activity and a very detailed profile of work on the ward.

To illustrate the value of this method, the following four findings are examples which emerged from an activity analysis collecting the information described above.

1. The failure to organise work in such a way that learners worked where possible with trained staff, led to a considerable loss of potentially valuable learning experience. Typically nurses worked with their peers in rank and age.
2. Only 46.5 per cent of nurses' time was spent in direct patient care. A total of 37 per cent of time was spent in direct contact with the patient.
3. Minimal amounts of overt teaching or learning were observed – of all ward activity only two per cent was devoted to this. Of this tiny proportion of educational activity less than a quarter was patient centred.
4. Consultants took up 11 per cent of sisters' time on average. This is lower than would have been predicted on sisters' own accounts of this part of their job.

For a full account of an application of activity analysis, and a sample form for recording the information see Reid (1986).

Activity analysis is carried out by one observer in a ward. It becomes tiring, so a relief observer is needed. But with the investment of two people, a massive amount of invaluable information becomes available. The method is very flexible in that it can be used to describe any aspect of ward activity which is of interest to the researcher.

Summary

It would be impossible in one chapter to provide even an overview of all the research techniques employed in nursing research. Instead this chapter has concentrated on providing some detail on the most useful and commonly used techniques and also on some little used but potentially very valuable techniques. We hope that we have offered a way forward for most types of nursing research project, but there are of course gaps. Participant and non-participant observation, for example, have not been explicitly covered, but clinical trials could be an example of either. Techniques which require a lot of funding or human resources have been excluded because this book has been written for the practising nurse who wants to do some work related research but does not have a great deal of time or resources at her disposal.

The research methods we have discussed will result in the collection of a great deal of information which has somehow to be presented in a form that is intelligible and meaningful to the reader. The next three chapters deal with the analysis of the data collected and the presentation of the results.

4

How to Describe and Summarise Data

Variables and their measurement

Much of the application of statistics is concerned with variation. The fact that variation exists makes statistics both necessary and desirable. For, if everyone was the same height or had the same blood pressure or held the same opinions, we would have no need of elaborate measurements and analysis. Statistics is therefore concerned in the main with *variables*. A variable can be defined as anything which may change in quantity or quality from one observation to the next observation. Examples would be height, weight, length of service or age.

There are two main types of variable – *discrete* and *continuous*. For example, the number of children in a family might be 3 or 4 but not 3.5, thus this variable takes discrete values. Weight, on the other hand might be 140 pounds or 141 pounds or anything in between, so weight is a continuous variable.

Levels of measurement

Variables are measured to provide the data on which the statistician will work. There are various levels of measurement. The lowest level of measurement is *nominal*, and this entails merely placing the subject in a category. For instance speciality is a nominal variable and medical, surgical, paediatric, or geriatric would be categories in a study of hospital patients. The next level of measurement is *ordinal*, and this entails placing the subject in ranked categories, for example grade would be a variable with ordinal categories, staff nurse, sister, nursing officer, senior nursing officer. The *interval* level of measurement gives numerical values to each measurement, such as height, blood pressure, pulse. The differences between these three levels of measurement may be summarised as follows.

1. Nominal measurement identifies differences in category.
2. Ordinal measurement identifies differences in category and differences in rank.
3. Interval measurement identifies differences in category and differences in rank and differences in amount.

It is important to consider the appropriate level of measurement before collecting data. For example, age is a variable that could be collected at either ordinal or interval level. It can be collected at ordinal level by asking people to tick the age category which applies:

Age	Tick as appropriate
0–15	
16–30	
31–45	
46–60	
61 or over	

For many studies this level of measurement of age is perfectly adequate. It may well be unnecessary to know the exact age and people will sometimes be reluctant to reveal this in any case! If the exact age is needed, however, you are collecting the data at interval level.

The level of measurement will determine the extent and nature of the analysis of the data. It is important to think about the analysis you wish to carry out when deciding on levels of measurement.

Population and sample

The totality of all possible observations of a variable is called the **population**. In practice it is rarely possible to include all of these in a study, so we look at a **sample**. There are a number of methods of sampling, one of which is simple random sampling, which ensures that each member of the population has an equal chance of being selected for the sample. The study is then based on the sample, but inferences about the entire population can be made on the basis of what is discovered about the sample. For this to be valid it is obviously essential that the sample is representative of the population. A correct sampling method should provide a representative sample, and in Chapter 3 the main sampling techniques which are used in nursing research are described.

Having obtained a representative sample, a number of variables will typically be measured on that sample. The average questionnaire, for example, will provide information on fifty or sixty variables. If 100 subjects have completed the questionnaire there will be in total some 5000 to 6000 pieces of information! The purpose of this chapter is to provide techniques for reducing and summarising the information provided by one variable.

This is often the first step in analysing a set of data. Each variable is taken one at a time. At this stage we are not interested in the relationship between variables. The following two chapters deal with that. The objective is to describe in summary form the information provided through the measurement of each individual variable. To illustrate the techniques, we will use two data sets, one a discrete variable and the other a continuous variable. The discrete variable is the number of occupied beds in a ward and the continuous variable is length of service in years at appointment to the ward sister/charge nurse grade. These are both interval level measurements. As we proceed through the techniques of reduction and summary we will indicate when these are appropriate for nominal and ordinal levels of measurements.

Pictorial representation

The use of pictorial or graphical representation is strongly recommended as a first step in describing a set of measurements on a variable. It provides an attractive and easily understood way of presenting information. The raw data on our two variables is as follows.

Variable 1 Number of occupied beds in a 30-bed unit on twenty occasions (sample of size 20).

> 28, 26, 23, 29, 29, 27, 27, 28, 26, 25, 26, 28, 30, 27, 25, 29, 27, 29, 30, 30

This is a discrete variable.

Variable 2 Length of service (years) on appointment to the ward sister/charge nurse grade for thirty sisters (sample of size 30).

> 1.6, 2.2, 6.1, 4.2, 5.1, 3.1, 2.2, 4.4, 6.2, 5.2, 3.2, 1.9, 3.3, 5.2, 6.2, 4.5, 2.4, 3.4, 5.4, 6.4, 4.5, 2.7, 4.6, 5.5, 3.4, 3.6, 3.9, 5.5, 4.6, 2.8

This is a continuous variable.

Pie chart

Each of these variables may be pictorially represented by a pie chart. This is a circular diagram divided into slices to represent the frequency with which particular values of the variable occur.

Variable 1 Number of occupied beds in a 30-bed unit.

For variable 1 which is discrete, the first step is to identify the discrete values which occur and to write these in order in a column. Only values which actually occur are represented in this table.

Values

23
25
26
27
28
29
30

Then beside each value which occurred we write down the frequency with which it occurred. For example, 23 occurred once, 25 occurred twice and so on. This will give

Values	Frequency
23	1
25	2
26	3
27	4
28	3
29	4
30	3
Total	20

Note that the total of the frequencies should be the sample size which was 20. The percentage frequency of each value is then calculated as follows.

$$\% \text{ frequency of the value } 25 = \frac{\text{frequency}}{\text{total frequency}} \times 100$$

$$= \frac{2}{20} \times 100 = 10\%$$

Repeating this for each value will give:

Value	Frequency	% Frequency
23	1	5
25	2	10
26	3	15
27	4	20
28	3	15
29	4	20
30	3	15
	20	100

Note that the total of the percentage frequencies should be 100%. The next step is to cut slices in a circular pie corresponding to the percentage frequencies. There are altogether 360 degrees in a circle, so to find the number of degrees corresponding to each percentage frequency:

$$\text{degrees corresponding to 10\% frequency} = 10\% \text{ of } 360$$
$$= \frac{10}{100} \times 360$$
$$= 36 \text{ degrees.}$$

Repeating this for each percentage frequency will give:

Value	Frequency	% Frequency	Degrees
23	1	5	18
25	2	10	36
26	3	15	54
27	4	20	72
28	3	15	54
29	4	20	72
30	3	15	54
	20	100	360

Using a protractor to measure out the degrees, the pie chart can now be drawn (Fig. 4.1).

It is now possible to see at a glance how frequent each level of bed occupancy was, relative to the others.

Variable 2 Length of service on appointment to ward sister/charge nurse grade.

This procedure is now repeated for the continuous variable. There is only one additional step which is that we place the data in groups before we begin. It is obvious that this is necessary since no individual value will tend to occur more than once in the data set.

Values

1.6, 2.2, 6.1, 4.2, 5.1, 3.1, 2.2, 4.4, 6.2, 5.2, 3.2, 1.9, 3.3, 5.2, 6.2,
4.5, 2.4, 3.4, 5.4, 6.4, 4.5, 2.7, 4.6, 5.5, 3.4, 3.6, 3.9, 5.5, 4.6, 2.8

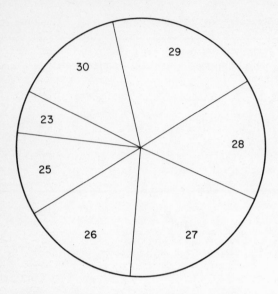

Fig. 4.1 Pie chart showing the frequency of the number of occupied beds in a 30 bed unit.

These observations are now placed in the following groups:

Length of service (years)

0–1
1.1–2
2.1–3
3.1–4
4.1–5
5.1–6
6.1–7

The choice of groups is arbitrary, but it is important to remember that the groups must be quite distinct from each other, with no overlap between groups. The groups must also be of equal range (i.e. equal interval length). The number of values which fall into each group, the group frequency, will now be shown. For example there were four values in the 6.1–7 group, 6.1, 6.2, 6.2 and 6.4.

Length of service (years)	Frequency
1.1–2	2
2.1–3	5
3.1–4	7
4.1–5	6
5.1–6	6
6.1–7	4
	30

We now proceed exactly as before to calculate the percentage frequency and the degrees. This will give:

Length of service (years)	Frequency	% Frequency	Degrees
1.1–2	2	7	25
2.1–3	5	17	61
3.1–4	7	23	83
4.1–5	6	20	72
5.1–6	6	20	72
6.1–7	4	13	47
	30	100	360

The pie chart will therefore be as shown in Fig. 4.2.

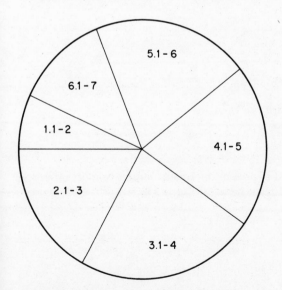

Fig. 4.2 Pie chart showing length of service on appointment to Ward Sister/Charge Nurse grade.

The immediate advantages of this simple technique are obvious. Compare the raw data set on variable 2, which conveys no real information whatever, with the pie chart which shows immediately the relative frequency with which the different ranges of values occurred. The pie chart conveys information at a glance.

The pie chart is also a good way of representing nominal or ordinal level data.

Other pictorial and graphical methods

Graphs
Simple graphs showing the score on a variable over time can be easily drawn. Figure 4.3 is an example of total daily workload for a ward (Barr's dependency method) over fourteen days.

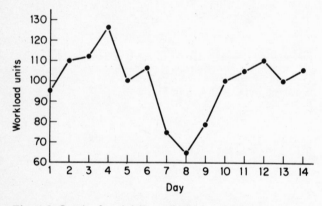

Fig. 4.3 Graph of total daily workload over 14 days.

Bar chart
A bar chart can be used to present information on the number of beds in Northern Ireland in different specialities as in Fig. 4.4.

Percentage component bar chart
A percentage component bar chart can be used to illustrate the components within a total. Figure 4.5 gives the percentage components of trained, learner and untrained nurses in three medical wards of a general hospital.

Histograms
The histogram provides the most commonly used method of representing the frequency with which each value occurs. This is called the frequency distribution. The first step is to tabulate the frequency of each value, for a

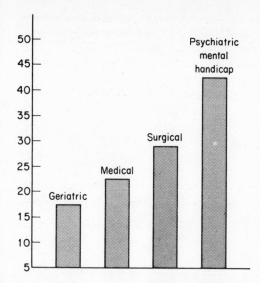

Fig. 4.4 Bar chart of number of beds in Northern Ireland in different specialities.

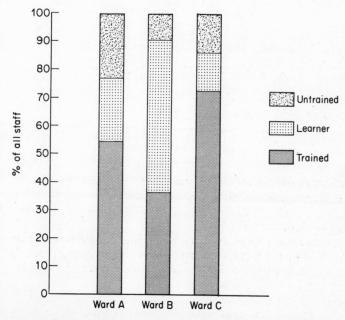

Fig. 4.5 Percentage component bar chart showing percentages of untrained, learner and trained nurses in three medical wards.

discrete variable, or the frequency of each range of values for a continuous variable. For our discrete variable, the number of occupied beds, we had:

Value	Frequency	% Frequency
23	1	5
25	2	10
26	3	15
27	4	20
28	3	15
29	4	20
30	3	15
	20	100

The histogram is drawn by plotting either frequency or percentage frequency against the values. Both are shown in Fig. 4.6.

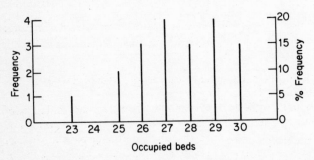

Fig. 4.6 Histogram showing frequency and percentage frequency of the number of occupied beds in a 30 bed unit.

Note that it is essential that the value 24 appears on the x-axis, even though there is zero frequency for this value.

For a continuous variable like length of service a similar approach is used, but blocks representing the frequency of each range are used rather than lines as in the discrete case to represent the frequency of each value. Figure 4.7 gives the histogram for length of service at appointment to the ward sister grade.

Length of service	Frequency	% Frequency
1.1–2	2	7
2.1–3	5	17
3.1–4	7	23
4.1–5	6	20
5.1–6	6	20
6.1–7	4	13
	30	100

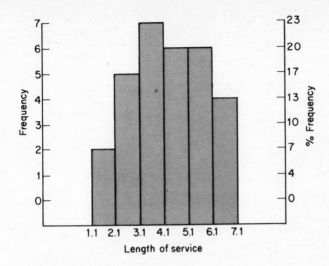

Fig. 4.7 Histogram of the length of serviçe at appointment to Ward Sister/Charge Nurse grade.

By inspection of these histograms, summary information about the variable is available.

It is possible to tell at a glance that the most frequent category for length of service is 3.1–4 years and that the average is likely to be around 4 years. The end points of the range of values are immediately identifiable and you can see whether the distribution is symmetrical around a middle point or whether it tails off to the right or the left. The term distribution refers to the spread of frequencies across values of a variable. These observations are important in the next stage of analysis which is the calculation of summary statistics to describe the distribution.

The value of pictorial representation of data cannot be over emphasised, and this section has covered only some of the available methods. There are others which would be equally appropriate.

Summary statistics

The next task is to calculate some numbers which will summarise the information which has just been represented as a frequency distribution. Most people will understand intuitively the usefulness of having an average for the range of values. In statistics we call an average a ***measure of location*** – but is it enough?

Consider one of the best known types of distribution, the symmetrical bell-shaped distribution. Such variables as height and weight have this kind of frequency distribution. Let us say that for some imaginary variable the average was 50. Does this adequately describe the distribution? Consider

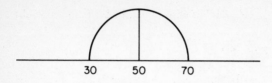

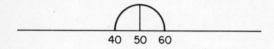

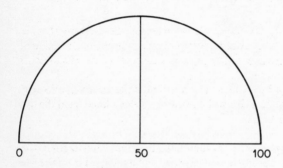

Fig. 4.8 Distributions.

Fig. 4.8. All of the distributions in this figure have an average of 50, but they are clearly very different types of distribution. What is required is a further summary measure to represent *scatter*, because the factor which distinguishes the three distributions is the extent to which the data are scattered or dispersed around the average. This second summary statistic is called a *measure of scatter* or a *measure of dispersion*.

For every distribution, therefore, the basic set of summary statistics comprises a measure of location and a measure of scatter. There are a number of different ways of measuring location and scatter, and the correct way will depend to some extent on the shape of the distribution.

Measures of location

The mean
The best known measure of location is the *mean*. This is the sum of all observations of the variable divided by the number of observations. For

example for our variable on the number of occupied beds the mean would be:

$$\frac{\begin{array}{c} 28 + 26 + 23 + 29 + 29 + 27 + 27 + \\ 28 + 26 + 25 + 26 + 28 + 30 + 27 + \\ 25 + 29 + 27 + 29 + 30 + 30 \end{array}}{20} = \frac{549}{20} = 27.45$$

A quicker way of calculating the mean would be from the frequency table. The mean is the sum of each value multiplied by its frequency divided by the number of observations

$$\frac{\begin{array}{c} (23 \times 1) + (25 \times 2) + (26 \times 3) + (27 \times 4) + (28 \times 3) + \\ (29 \times 4) + (30 \times 3) \end{array}}{20}$$

$$= \frac{23 + 50 + 78 + 108 + 84 + 116 + 90}{20} = \frac{549}{20} = 27.45$$

Either way, the answer is 27.45 beds. It is always worth checking that the answer looks sensible. It would not be possible, for example, for a mean to be smaller than the smallest value or larger than the largest value. It should lie somewhere around the middle.

For a continuous variable, the mean is calculated in the same way. You can check that for the length of service variable the mean calculated from the raw data is 123.3/30 = 4.11 years.

Calculating the mean of group data Sometimes data is collected in groups or, as in the case of the length of service variable, it can be grouped from the raw data.

Values	Frequency
1.1–2	2
2.1–3	5
3.1–4	7
4.1–5	6
5.1–6	6
6.1–7	4
	30

While it is perfectly feasible to calculate the length of service mean in the usual way from the raw data, the above grouped data will serve to illustrate the method of calculation of the mean of grouped data. Length of service is now being treated as if the data had been collected in the above groups.

For each group the mid-point is found. This is 1.55 for the first group ((1.1 + 2)/2) and for the other groups 2.55, 3.55, 4.55, 5.55 and 6.55 respectively. The mean is now calculated by finding the sum of each mid-point multiplied by its frequency and divided by the number of observations.

$$\frac{\begin{array}{c}(2 \times 1.55) + (5 \times 2.55) + (7 \times 3.55) + \\ (6 \times 4.55) + (6 \times 5.55) + (4 \times 6.55)\end{array}}{30} = \frac{127.5}{30} = 4.25 \text{ years}$$

This is the only method for calculating the mean if the data is collected in groups. If you have the raw data and then group it, you will lose accuracy by calculating the mean using the grouped formula. In the above case the correct mean is 4.11. The grouped method gives a mean of 4.25 which is slightly inaccurate. The grouped method should only be used if the raw data is not available, or if there are so many observations on the raw data that it will save a substantial amount of time to use the grouped method.

Two formulae have now been used, although the formulae have not yet been stated explicitly. The mean is usually written $\bar{x}$, where x represents the variable

$$\bar{x} = \frac{\Sigma x}{n} = \frac{\text{sum of all observations}}{\text{number of observations}}$$

The symbol Σx means that all the x values are added together (i.e. all the observations of the variable, x). The symbol, n, is usually used to represent the number of observations or the sample size.

If each individual x value occurs f times, the formula becomes

$$\bar{x} = \frac{\Sigma fx}{n}$$

and this is the formula used above to find the sum of each value multiplied by its frequency and then divided by the total number of observations.

The median

Another measure of location is the ***median***. The median is that observation with the same number of observations smaller than it as larger than it. In other words, when the observations are ranked the median is the middle observation. For an odd number of ranked observations, there is one number which is the median. For example, for 21 observations in rank order the median is the eleventh which has ten observations below it and ten above it. For an even number of ranked observations the median is the average of the two in the middle. For example, for 40 observations in rank order the median is the average of the twentieth and the twenty-first observations.

For our variable, the number of occupied beds, the rank order is as follows:

23, 25, 25, 26, 26, 26, 27, 27, 27, 27, 28, 28, 28, 29, 29, 29, 29, 30, 30, 30

The median is the average of the tenth and eleventh;

$$\frac{27 + 28}{2} = 27.5$$

For our variable on length of service at appointment to the sister/charge nurse grade, the rank order is as follows:

1.6, 1.9, 2.2, 2.2, 2.4, 2.7, 2.8, 3.1, 3.2, 3.3, 3.4, 3.4, 3.6, 3.9, 4.2,
4.4, 4.5, 4.5, 4.6, 4.6, 5.1, 5.2, 5.2, 5.4, 5.5, 5.5, 6.1, 6.2, 6.2, 6.4

The median is the average of the fifteenth and sixteenth values;

$$\frac{4.2 + 4.4}{2} = 4.3$$

Calculating the median of group data For discrete data presented in groups, like the number of occupied beds, the median may be quickly found by first calculating the **cumulative frequency** of each value. The cumulative frequency of a value is the frequency of that value plus the frequency of all smaller values. Thus, for our variable, number of occupied beds:

Value	Frequency	Cumulative frequency
23	1	1
25	2	3
26	3	6
27	4	10
28	3	13
29	4	17
30	3	20

So there are 10 values of 27 or below, 13 values of 28 or below and so on.

From the cumulative frequency it can be seen that the tenth ordered value is 27 and the eleventh ordered value is 28 and the median is therefore 27.5, as before.

The data on length of service will be treated as if they had been collected in the following form:

Groups (values)	Frequency	Cumulative frequency
1.1–2	2	2
2.1–3	5	7
3.1–4	7	14
4.1–5	6	20
5.1–6	6	26
6.1–7	4	30

The median is the average of the fifteenth and sixteenth ordered observations. Since the first 14 ordered observations take us up to the end of the third group (3.1–4) it is clear that the fifteenth and sixteenth ordered observations are the first two observations in the fourth group (4.1–5). If the exact values of those observations are known, the exact median can be calculated.

If the exact values are not known, for instance if we know only that 6 observations lie between 4.1 and 5.0, the values can be estimated on the assumption that the six observations are spread evenly across the group. So the first observations in the class (the fifteenth ordered observation) will be one sixth of the class width into the group. The estimate is therefore 4.1 + (1/6 × 0.9) = 4.25. The second observation into the class (the sixteenth ordered observation) will be two sixths of the class width into the group. The estimate is therefore 4.1 + (2/6 × 0.9) = 4.4. So the median will be the average of 4.25 and 4.4, which is 4.325. Note that this method should only be used when the exact values are not known.

The mode
A final measure of location is the **mode**. This is the value which occurs most often in the data set, that is the value with the highest frequency. For the variable, number of occupied beds, there are two modes, 27 and 29 which each occur four times. A distribution with two modes is called **bimodal**, but it is more usual to find a single mode. If a continuous variable like length of service is grouped, the model group is the one with the greatest frequency.

Selection of appropriate measure of location
Three measures of location have now been described. In practice the mean and the median are the most common used. Depending on the shape of the distribution one or other should be selected. The only instance in which it does not matter whether the mean or the median is calculated is if the distribution is symmetrical and bell-shaped, as in Fig. 4.9. In this instance the mean and the median will be equal.

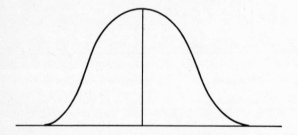

Fig. 4.9 A symmetrical bell-shaped distribution.

Otherwise, it is recommended that the median be used, especially for skewed distributions. A skewed distribution is one with a long tail to the right or the left (Fig. 4.10). The distribution in Fig. 4.10a has a long tail to the right. This means that there is a very small number of very high values. In such a case, the mean will be distorted by the very high values and will not represent the data as a whole. The long tail will tend to pull the mean towards it. The median, on the other hand, is not affected by the extreme values and will give a good measure of central tendency.

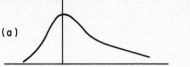 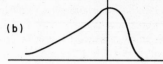

Fig. 4.10 Skewed distributions.

Measures of dispersion

Along with a measure of location, a measure of dispersion is needed to describe the distribution of a variable. The mean has a partner, the standard deviation, which measures scatter, and the partner of the median is the semi-interquartile range.

The standard deviation

The standard deviation is a measure of the average dispersion of the variable. Consider a variable, x, with a symmetrical distribution and a mean of $\bar{x}$ where x is any other value of the variable. The scatter or dispersion of x from the mean, $\bar{x}$, could be described simply by the distance between x and $\bar{x}$ $(x - \bar{x})$. This distance could be calculated for every value of x and all the distances added together to obtain a measure of the total scatter of the variable. This measure could be written

$$\Sigma(x - \bar{x})$$

which is the sum of the distances of each point from the mean. The problem is that because the mean is the central point, the various $(x - \bar{x})$ components will cancel each other out and the sum will be zero. To avoid this problem, the square of each distance is used, i.e. $(x - \bar{x})^2$. This means that the negative distances (where x lies to the left of $\bar{x}$) become positive when squared, so each x contributes a positive component to the total scatter, its squared distance from the mean. The total scatter is then $\Sigma(x - \bar{x})^2$. Obviously the size of this total scatter will depend on the number of observations. The measure $\Sigma(x - \bar{x})^2$ will be very much bigger for a data set of size 100, each contributing a component, than for a data set of size 10. So an averaging factor is needed. Dividing $\Sigma(x - \bar{x})^2$ by n − 1, where n is the size of the data set, provides a measure of the average squared distance from the mean. (Within the scope of this text the correct divisor is n − 1. The reason why it is n − 1 rather than n lies beyond the scope of this text, but any standard statistical textbook can be consulted for the explanation.) The distances earlier were squared to avoid terms cancelling each other out, so a square root is now taken to obtain the average distance from the mean. So the standard deviation (S) is

$$S = \sqrt{\frac{\Sigma(x - \bar{x})^2}{n - 1}}$$

This formula could now be used, but there is an equivalent and very much easier version of it to use in practice. This is

$$S = \sqrt{\frac{\Sigma x^2 - \frac{(\Sigma x)^2}{n}}{n - 1}}$$

where Σx^2 = the sum of the squares of each observation,
$(\Sigma x)^2$ = the square of the sum of the observations, and
n = the sample size.

If for example, we wanted to calculate the standard deviation of a small set of data on family size, 2, 3, 4, 5

x	x²	
2	4	
3	9	
4	16	n = 4
5	25	
14	54	

so in the formula

$$S = \sqrt{\frac{\Sigma x^2 - \frac{(\Sigma x)^2}{n}}{n - 1}} = \sqrt{\frac{54 - \frac{(14)^2}{4}}{4 - 1}}$$

$$= \sqrt{\frac{54 - \frac{196}{4}}{3}}$$

$$= 1.29$$

Calculating this on the variable, number of occupied beds, we have:

x	x²
23	529
25	625
25	625
26	676
26	676
26	676
27	729
27	729
27	729
27	729
28	784
28	784

$$S = \sqrt{\frac{15139 - \frac{(549)^2}{20}}{19}}$$

x	x^2
28	784
29	841
29	841
29	841
29	841
30	900
30	900
30	900
549	15139

= 1.905

A short cut to the standard deviation and the mean   There is a short cut which can be used in calculating a standard deviation if the data can be reduced to simple small numbers by subtracting the same number from each observation. For instance, we could subtract 23 from every observation in the previous example on occupied beds, and calculate the standard deviation on the smaller numbers:

x	x
0	0
2	4
2	4
3	9
3	9
3	9
4	16
4	16
4	16
4	16
5	25
5	25
5	25
6	36
6	36
6	36
6	36
7	49
7	49
7	49
89	465

$$S = \sqrt{\frac{\Sigma x^2 - \frac{(\Sigma x)^2}{n}}{n - 1}}$$

$$S = \sqrt{\frac{465 - \frac{89^2}{20}}{19}}$$

= 1.905

You can see that the answer is exactly the same, but the arithmetic a good deal less taxing.

A similar short cut can be used to calculate the mean number of occupied beds. Again, subtract a constant, (23 in this example) from each observation and find the mean of the smaller numbers. Call this the adjusted mean

$$\text{adjusted mean} = \frac{\text{sum of smaller numbers}}{\text{number of observations}} = \frac{89}{20} = 4.45$$

Then add the constant back on to the adjusted mean

mean = adjusted mean plus constant
= 4.45 + 23
= 27.45

Check that this is the same answer as was obtained by the conventional calculation of the mean, earlier in this chapter.

The standard deviation and mean of the variable, length of service at appointment to sister, could be calculated in exactly the same ways. The correct answers are 1.40 for the standard deviation and 4.11 for the mean.

The standard deviation for grouped data　When data are presented in groups and the exact values are not known, a different form of the formula for the standard deviation may be used. The grouped data on age at appointment (although the raw figures are available in this case) will serve to illustrate the method.

Group range	Frequency (f)	Mid-point (x)	fx	x^2	fx^2
1.1–2	2	1.55	3.10	2.403	4.806
2.1–3	5	2.55	12.75	6.503	32.515
3.1–4	7	3.55	24.85	12.603	88.221
4.1–5	6	4.55	27.30	20.703	124.218
5.1–6	6	5.55	33.30	30.803	184.818
6.1–7	4	6.55	26.20	42.903	171.612
			127.50		606.190

the standard deviation is given by

$$\sqrt{\frac{\Sigma fx^2 - \dfrac{(\Sigma fx)^2}{n}}{n-1}}$$

Σfx^2 is the sum of the products of each mid-point squared and its frequency (see final column of preceding table).

Σfx^2 = $(2 \times 2.403) + (5 \times 6.503) + (7 \times 12.603) + (6 \times 20.703) + (6 \times 30.803) + (4 \times 42.903)$
= 606.19

Σfx is the sum of the products of each mid point and its frequency (see fourth column of preceding table).

$$\Sigma fx = (2 \times 1.55) + (5 \times 2.55) + (7 \times 3.55) + (6 \times 4.55) +$$
$$(6 \times 5.55) + (4 \times 6.55)$$
$$= 127.5$$

so the standard deviation is

$$\sqrt{\frac{606.19 - \dfrac{127.5^2}{30}}{29}} = 1.489$$

This is an approximation based on the assumption that every observation in the range takes the mid-point value. Obviously if the actual values of each observation are known, the grouped method should preferably not be used since there is a loss of accuracy. For the above example the true standard deviation was 1.397, and the value obtained using the grouped method was 1.489. However, the grouped method is the only possibility, when individual values are not available, and is also used sometimes to save time with very large raw data sets.

Finally, it should be noted that the variance is another commonly used measure of scatter. The variance is simply the square of the standard deviation. In the above example the variance is $(1.489)^2 = 2.217$.

The semi-interquartile range

The *semi-interquartile range* is the measure of scatter of dispersion which partners the median. Like the median, it operates on an ordered data set. The median was the value which chopped the data set in half. Look for two further cut-off points, the one which cuts off the bottom quarter of the data, which is called Q_1 and the one which cuts off the top quarter, which is called Q_3 (see Fig. 4.11). The semi-interquartile range is given by $\frac{1}{2}(Q_3 - Q_1)$.

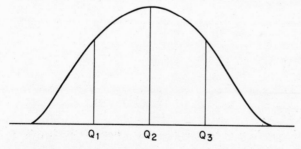

Fig. 4.11 Quartiles.

Applying this to the example on occupied beds, where there were twenty ordered observations:

23, 25, 25, 26, 26, 26, 27, 27, 27, 27, 28, 28, 28, 29, 29, 29, 29, 30, 30, 30

We want a value, Q_1 which cuts off the bottom five and another value Q_3 which cuts off the top five. Since we have twenty observations, averaging the fifth and sixth will produce a number which cuts off the bottom five. So Q_1 = $\frac{1}{2}(26 + 26)$ = 26. Averaging the fifteenth and sixteenth will produce a number which cuts off the top five. So $Q_3 = \frac{1}{2}(29 + 29)$ = 29. So the semi-interquartile range (SIQR) is $\frac{1}{2}(29 - 26)$ = 1.5.

Repeating this on the data on length of service would give a value for Q_1 of $\frac{1}{2}(2.8 + 3.1)$ = 2.95, and a value of Q_3 of $\frac{1}{2}(5.2 + 5.4)$ = 5.3. So the SIQR = $\frac{1}{2}(5.3 - 2.95)$ = 1.175.

If the data are grouped, a technique analogous to that described for the calculation of the median for grouped data can be used (page 63). You can use the grouped data on length of service to illustrate this. You should find that Q_1 = 3.114 and Q_3 = 5.625 so the SIQR is 1.256.

Summary

This chapter has traced a path from the mass of raw data to concise pictorial representation and statistical summary. For every variable there is a choice of pictorial methods, some of which we have described. This is an important first stage in describing the variable.

The next stage is to calculate two summary measures, a measure of location and a measure of scatter. If the data set is symmetrical you can choose either the mean with the standard deviation *or* the median with the semi-interquartile range. If the data distribution is skewed, calculation of the median and the SIQR represents the best choice of measures.

Whichever measures are selected the original set of data has been reduced to two meaningful numbers representing location and scatter. This is a neat illustration of our belief that the purpose of statistics is to simplify, not to make life more difficult.

5

Inference and Hypothesis Testing

Statistical inference

The previous chapter concentrated on the use of statistics in describing data. These statistics have related to descriptions of the data in hand; to the subjects for which information was available, but the subjects in hand might well be a sample from a larger population. So a question is raised about the extent to which we can generalise about the whole population, rather than simply describe the sample which has been measured and on which the calculations are based. The process of making generalisations about the wider population from the results on the sample is called statistical inference.

Chapter 4 examined data on length of service at appointment to ward sister/charge nurse grade from a sample of size 30. What inferences can be made from this sample to the wider population?

Assume that the sample was drawn from a list of all appointments to ward sister in the Westwick Regional Health Authority in 1985. The distribution for all the appointments made in the Authority could be illustrated by Fig. 5.1. The mean of the population is referred to as μ (mu), and its standard deviation σ (sigma). The use of random sampling allows inferences to be made about the population as a whole from data collected on the sample.

The histogram based on the sample looked like Fig. 5.2. The mean of the sample, was $\bar{x} = 4.11$ and the standard deviation was $S = 1.4$. The sample mean $\bar{x}$ is an estimate of the population mean, μ. That is, the fact that the sample mean was 4.11 enables the inference to be made that the mean age at appointment for all sisters in the Region in 1985 was 4.11. Similarly we can make the inference that the standard deviation for the population of all appointments to sister in the Region in 1985 was 1.4. Because the sample was randomly collected, we are able to go beyond the calculation of descriptive sample statistics and make two valid inferences about the population.

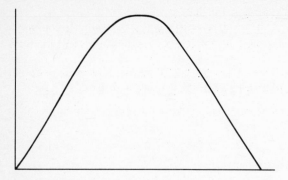

Fig. 5.1 Distribution of length of service at appointment to Ward Sister.

Note that it would not be strictly valid to make any inference about the mean age of appointment in any other health authority, or in this health authority in any year other than 1985. Inferences should strictly be limited to the population from which the sample is drawn. Of course, common sense may well suggest that wider inference would be valid, but there are no statistical grounds for this.

A number of further interesting questions now arise.

1. From a national data source it is known that the average length of service at appointment to sister is 5.5 years for all UK nurses. Is the Westwick average of 4.11 different enough to suggest that something different is

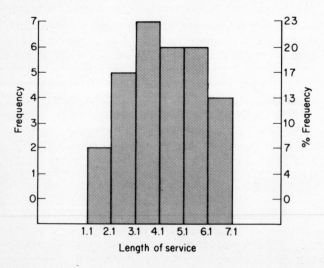

Fig. 5.2 Histogram from example of length of service at appointment to Ward Sister.

happening in the Westwick Region?

2. A similar sample could be collected from the Eastwick Region and a mean of 3.25 calculated. Is this Region significantly different from Westwick?

3. The sample collected in Westwick was all female. If we were to collect data on a sample of males, would the average be different?

To answer such questions, we need to apply inferential techniques called tests of significance.

Use of tests of significance

Tests of significance are used to establish whether certain inferences can be made, and if so, with what probability of being correct. If may well be worth explaining in a little more detail the meaning of the term 'tests of significance'.

Consider again the example above, where the question of a difference in mean lengths of service for males and females arose. If samples of data are collected for males and females and means calculated, it is highly unlikely that these sample means would ever be exactly equal, in practice. One would intuitively accept that a small difference could well be consistent with there being no real difference between men and women's average length of service. The key question is when is a difference big enough to be statistically significant? Tests of significance are designed to detect genuine or 'significant' effects as distinct from small effects which are simply due to variation in the data collected on the samples from the whole population.

A significance test cannot establish conclusions with certainty, so should never be interpreted in a 'black or white' manner. A significance test can however establish conclusions with a known probability of error. For example, it might be concluded that males and females have different average lengths of service with a 5% chance of error. The probability or degree of certainty that the conclusion is wrong is 1 in 20 (5%). All significance tests provide conclusions with stated probabilities of error.

The logic of significance testing
There is a simple logic which underlies every significance test. To illustrate these steps, the example of whether the average length of service of the Westwick population (inferred from the sample) is different from national length of service will be used.

Step 1 State the null hypothesis.
In carrying out tests of statistical significance a null hypothesis should always be explicitly stated. A null hypothesis is not necessarily the same as the research hypothesis. A research hypothesis is a statement of the anticipated finding based on the theoretical background to the study. A null hypothesis is one which states an assumption of null effect which is then to

be statistically tested and then accepted as true or rejected as false. For the example on length of service, there are four possible hypotheses which could be stated prior to data collection.

1. The Westwick population average differs from the national average.
2. The Westwick population average is less than the national average.
3. The Westwick population average is greater than the national average.
4. The Westwick population average does not differ from the national average.

Only the fourth statement is a null hypothesis in that it specifies no difference. The first three statements could be described as research hypotheses, but only the fourth is a null hypothesis which is the hypothesis to be tested by the statistical test.

Step 2   Collect the data. In this case the data collected would be from the sample of size 30 randomly selected from all Westwick appointments in 1985.

Step 3   Calculate a test statistic which will give you the probability of observing the data you collected, *if the null hypothesis is true*. This test statistic depends on the kind of significance test being carried out. Detail of the calculation of individual test statistics will be provided with each test described later in this chapter.

Step 4   If the data collected had a high probability of occurring, assuming the null hypothesis were true as indicated by the statistical test performed, accept the null hypothesis, that is, conclude that there is no difference between the Westwick average and the national average. If the data collected had a low probability of occurrence under the null hypothesis, reject the null hypothesis. In this case you would accept one of the alternative hypotheses stated under Step 1. The level of probability at which the null hypothesis would be rejected varies according to the type of study being undertaken and is set *before* carrying out the statistical test. A level of probability of 5% or less ($P < 5\%$) is commonly taken as an appropriate level in much of the nursing research carried out.

Tests of significance

In the remainder of this chapter a range of significance tests using these steps is described. Particular emphasis is placed on the null hypothesis, listing the data collected, showing the detail of the calculation of the test statistics and the conclusion of the test.

Selection of tests

A question which often arises in the mind of the student of statistics is how to select a test. Any textbook will provide a confusing plethora of tests. This book covers only a selection of tests, but it may be helpful to provide a framework for the selection of tests and an indication of where those selected for this text are placed within that framework.

The first two questions to be asked are:

1. Do you need a one sample or a two sample test?
2. Do you wish to use a parametric or a non-parametric (N-P) technique?

Answering the first question in simple. If you are testing a hypothesis involving one sample on one variable you want a one sample test. If you will be collecting two samples of data and your hypothesis involves comparing a variable across both populations, a two sample test will be needed. It is, of course, possible to generate hypotheses involving more than two populations. This is the realm of multi-variate analysis and beyond the scope of this text and it is recommended that the help of a statistician be sought before attempting analysis of this kind. For our present purposes, therefore, a one sample or two sample test will be adequate.

The second question hangs on whether the data come from a known distribution (with known parameters, when you can use a parametric test) or whether the distribution is not known, in which case you should use a non-parametric test. It may be helpful to describe briefly one of the best known distributions.

The Normal distribution
The best known is probably the Normal or Gaussian distribution. Height and weight are examples of variables with this distributional form, which is bell-shaped and symmetrical. A good deal of classical statistical theory was based on the Normal distribution, so some of the statistical tests in this chapter require this form of distribution. Some variables, such as height, are known to have a Normal distribution within the general population. The problem in applying the techniques which follow is in deciding whether the use of a method requiring a Normal distribution is justified when the underlying distribution is not known.

Full testing for Normality without access to a computer is time-consuming and difficult. We suggest that you either seek computing assistance or use a rule-of-thumb procedure. Draw up a histogram for your sample. If (a) the variable is continuous and (b) the shape of the distribution is approximately bell-shaped and symmetrical, you may reasonably assume that your variable is Normally distributed. Otherwise, use a non-parametric test.

Non-parametric tests
Non-parametric tests are usually easier to carry out than parametric tests. The main disadvantage is that they tend to be less sensitive and less powerful than parametric tests. However, they are very suitable for the testing of simple hypotheses, and in general non-parametric tests are more suitable for the kinds of data generated by nursing research. Survey data, for example, being mostly discrete variables, often measured by ranking scales, will not

be Normally distributed. So we would recommend that in many instances a non-parametric technique will be appropriate.

Classification of significance tests used in this text

Table 5.1 provides a helpful classification of the significance tests which follow in terms of the two factors just discussed. For a fuller range of non-parametric tests we would recommend Sidney Seigel's book on *Nonparametric Statistics for the Behavioural Sciences*, (1956) which, incidentally, contains a tabular summary similar to Table 5.1 for a much wider range of tests.

Table 5.1

	One sample	Two sample
Parametric	One sample t-test (interval)	Two sample paired t-test (interval) Two sample independent t-test (interval)
Non-parametric	Kolmogorov-Smirnov one sample test (ordinal) One sample chi-squared test (nominal)	McNemar test (paired, nominal) Wilcoxon signed-ranks test (paired, ordinal) Mann–Whitney test (independent, ordinal) χ^2 two sample test (independent, nominal)

One sample tests

Three examples of one sample tests follow, one parametric and two non-parametric. In each case the test is illustrated with an example, setting out the null hypothesis, the calculation of the test statistic and the conclusion. The level of measurement of data required for the test is also indicated.

The t-test

This is used to test whether a sample belongs to a distribution with a known mean. The t-test is valid for a variable with a Normal distribution, although it has been shown that where the t-test is used with minor deviations from the Normal distribution, the results are fairly valid. The t-test for this reason is described as *robust*, meaning relatively insensitive to departures from Normality. Nevertheless it should be remembered that the formal assumption when using this test is that the variable has a Normal distribution.

Example 1 Is the average length of service at appointment to ward sister/charge nurse in the Westwick Region the same as that for the whole of the UK (5.5 years)?

Step 1 The null hypothesis (NH) is that the average for the Westwick areas does not differ from the national average in age of appointment to ward sister/charge nurse.

Step 2 Collection of data on a sample of appointments in the Westwick Region. The sample of size 30 is:

1.6, 2.2, 6.1, 4.2, 5.1, 3.1, 2.2, 4.4, 6.2, 5.2, 3.2, 1.9, 3.3, 5.2, 6.2,
4.5, 2.4, 3.4, 5.4, 6.4, 4.5, 2.7, 4.6, 5.5, 3.4, 3.6, 3.9, 5.5, 5.5, 2.8

(N.B. This is the data used for variable 2 in the previous Chapter 4.)

Step 3 Calculation of the test statistic. The test statistic for a one sample t-test is

$$t = \frac{\bar{x} - \mu}{S/\sqrt{n}}$$

where $\bar{x}$ is the sample mean, S is the sample standard deviation, n is the sample size, and μ is the mean of the population against which we are testing the sample to see if it belongs.

So in this case $\bar{x} = 4.11$, $S = 1.40$, and $n = 30$. (These sample statistics were calculated in the previous chapter.)

Since we are testing whether the sample mean differs from the national mean, $\mu = 5.5$. So,

$$t = \frac{4.11 - 5.5}{1.40/\sqrt{30}} = -5.44.$$

The negative sign may be disregarded, giving a value for t of 5.44.

Step 4 The next task is to use the test statistic to deduce how likely it would be to obtain these data under the null hypothesis, that is, if it were correct that the Westwick average did not differ from the national average, how likely would the observed data be to occur? This is done by comparing the calculated t-statistic with a tabulated value obtained from standard tables. Table 1 in the Appendix gives a set of t-tables (we would recommend Neave's statistical tables (1981) which constitute a comprehensive set of tables for a wide range of significance tests).

The figure required from the table is that for $n - 1$ degrees of freedom and the 5% significance level. In this case, therefore, the appropriate t is that with 29 degrees of freedom at the 5% significance level. We write this as:

$$t_{29,5\%} = 2.0452$$

The number is found by tracing the row giving 29 degrees of freedom and the column giving the 5% significance level, and finding the number at the point of intersection of the appropriate row and column.

The tabulated value of t, 2.0452 is now compared with the number you have calculated, 5.44. The calculated t is greater, so you reject the null hypothesis at the 5% level. This means that you reject the null hypothesis with less than a 5% chance of error.

Thus the conclusion can be drawn that the Westwick Region differs from the national picture in length of service at appointment to ward sister/charge nurse.

You should be able to see intuitively how Step 4 works. If the Westwick area does not differ from the national picture you would expect $\bar{x}$ and μ to be very similar and $\bar{x} - \mu$ to be close to zero. Therefore the t-statistic which is $(\bar{x} - \mu)/(S\sqrt{n})$ should be very small. Very small is defined as smaller than the appropriate tabulated t-statistic, in which case you accept the null hypothesis. If Westwick *is* different from the national average, you would expect $\bar{x} - \mu$, and hence the t-statistic, to be large; larger than the tabulated t-statistic in which case you reject the null hypothesis of 'no difference'.

Example 2   Let us take another example. If, in fact, the UK average age at appointment to ward sister was only 4.3, does the Westwick Region differ from this?

Step 1   Null hypothesis. The Westwick Region does not differ from the UK in the age of appointment to ward sister/charge nurse.

Step 2   Data collection – same as in Example 1

Step 3

$$t = \frac{\bar{x} - \mu}{S/\sqrt{n}} = \frac{4.11 - 4.3}{1.40/\sqrt{30}} = -0.74$$

Take the positive value t = 0.74

Step 4   The tabulated statistic $t_{29,5\%} = 2.0452$. The calculated t is less than this so we accept the null hypothesis and conclude that the Westwick Region does not differ significantly from the UK in length of service at appointment to sister.

It should finally be noted that we have carried out what is called a two-tailed test in these examples, in that the conclusion related to establishing a difference in either direction. Had we initially wanted to look only at the research hypothesis that Westwick had a higher average length of service, a one-tailed test would have been carried out. This is different only at Step 4 in that a one-tailed tabulated t-statistic must be used (see Table 2 in the Appendix). Otherwise the procedure is the same.

The t-test is for interval level data. It cannot be used with ordinal or nominal data.

The Kolmogorov–Smirnov one sample test

This is a non-parametric test suitable for ordinal data. It is concerned with the degree of agreement between the distribution of a set of sample values and some specified theoretical distribution. It determines whether the scores in the sample can reasonably be thought to have come from a population having the theoretical distribution.

Example A mouthwash can be made up in varying degrees of salinity. Five mouth washes are made up in 1%, 2%, 3%, 4% and 5% saline solutions respectively. These are ranked one to five. Ten randomly selected patients are asked which they prefer. If the amount of saline is unimportant to the subjects, each rank should be chosen equally often. If the amount of saline is important, the subjects should consistently favour one of the extreme ranks.

Step 1 The null hypothesis is that the degree of salinity is not important to the subjects.

Step 2 Ten subjects are asked to state their preferences with the following results:

Rank of mouthwash	1	2	3	4	5
Number of subjects choosing that rank	0	1	0	5	4

Step 3 The calculation of the test statistic is as follows.

(a) If the saline is unimportant you would expect $\frac{1}{5}$ of the subjects to choose each rank.

Rank	1	2	3	4	5
Proportion choosing that rank under the NH	$\frac{1}{5}$	$\frac{1}{5}$	$\frac{1}{5}$	$\frac{1}{5}$	$\frac{1}{5}$

(b) Then calculate the cumulative proportions for each rank (the proportions choosing that rank or a lower rank, under the N.H.)

Rank	1	2	3	4	5
Cumulative proportion choosing that rank under NH	$\frac{1}{5}$	$\frac{2}{5}$	$\frac{3}{5}$	$\frac{4}{5}$	$\frac{5}{5}$

(c) Then calculate the cumulative proportions of the observed choices (from the data collected).

Rank	1	2	3	4	5
Cumulative proportion of observed choices	$\frac{0}{10}$	$\frac{1}{10}$	$\frac{1}{10}$	$\frac{6}{10}$	$\frac{10}{10}$

(d) Now calculate the difference between the proportions in (b) and (c) for each ranked pair and the test statistic, D, is the greatest difference. You can see that the greatest difference is $\frac{5}{10}$ for rank 3. So D = 5/10 = 0.5.

Step 4 Use Table 3 in the Appendix to see how to interpret the result. For a sample of size 10 the critical value is 0.410. The calculated D value is greater than this, so the null hypothesis is rejected at the 5% level of significance. The conclusion is that there are significant preferences about the salinity of mouthwashes among the study subjects.

This technique would be very useful in any small scale study of patient preferences where the choices can be ranked. The calculations are elementary.

The χ^2 (chi-squared) one sample test

Frequently the researcher is interested in the number of responses or subjects which fall into various categories. The purpose of the test is to establish whether the distribution observed differs from the distribution expected under the null hypothesis. This test can be used on nominal, ordinal or interval level data.

Example A nurse manager wishes to investigate whether wastage of qualified nurses in the hospital is speciality related.

Step 1 The null hypothesis is that there is no relationship between the wastage of qualified nurses and the speciality in which they worked.

Step 2 Collect data on a sample of all qualified nurse leavers for a period of one year, broken down by speciality. To simplify the calculations assume that there are equal numbers of nurses working in surgical, medical and other specialities. Results are as follows:

	Medicine	Surgery	Other	Total
Leavers	35	30	25	90

Step 3 Calculate the number you would expect in each category under the null hypothesis. If there is no relationship between wastage and speciality you would expect the 90 leavers to be equally distributed, 30 in each category. You now have for each category an observed number of leavers from your data (O) and the expected number of leavers under the null hypothesis (E). The test statistic is

$$\chi^2 = \Sigma \frac{(O - E)^2}{E}$$

For each category calculate the difference between the observed and expected value squared, divided by the expected value and add:

	O	E	O − E	(O − E)²	(O − E)²/E
Medicine	35	30	5	25	0.83
Surgery	30	30	0	0	0
Other	25	30	−5	25	0.83
					1.66

So the test statistic $\chi^2 = 1.66$.

Step 4 Now look up a tabulated value of χ^2 from statistical tables to interpret your result. Table 4 in the Appendix gives these values. To obtain the correct value trace the row with n – 1 degrees of freedom, where n is the number of categories you have used, which in this case is three. So, you want $\chi^2_{2,5\%}$ which is 5.991. The value calculated is smaller than the tabulated figure, which means the null hypothesis that there is no relationship between the speciality and the wastage of qualified nurses is accepted. Had the calculated figure been larger than 5.991 you would reject the null hypothesis at the 5% level, that is, with less than a 5% chance of being wrong.

Three kinds of one sample test have been described. They are not alternatives – it should be clear that they are geared to different kinds of hypotheses, different data distributions and different levels of measurement. They should, between them, offer a way forward for most hypotheses which you might want to test on a single sample.

Two sample tests

Two sample tests typically compare the means of the samples or some other sample statistics to investigate whether the samples come from the same distribution or are from different distributions. Two examples of parametric tests will be described, for use in quite distinct circumstances, and four examples of non-parametric tests. For each test, the level of measurement of the data will be indicated.

Two sample paired t-test
This test assumes that there are two equal sized samples of paired observations from populations with Normal distributions and that the standard deviations for the two distributions are equal. Paired observations in practice could be sets of two observations on the same subjects or sets of two readings from the same biochemical samples.

Example You want to know if there is any difference in temperature recordings measured in the mouth and in the axilla. You measure each of these on ten subjects to produce ten paired readings.

Step 1 The null hypothesis is that there is no difference between mouth and axillary temperature, i.e. the samples come from the same distribution.

Step 2 Axillary and mouth temperatures are taken on a sample of ten patients with the following results:

Patient	Mouth Temp (°F)	Axillary Temp (°F)
1	95	93
2	94	94
3	98	99
4	98	96
5	99	97

Patient	Mouth Temp (°F)	Axillary Temp (°F)
6	102	101
7	97	95
8	98	97
9	96	94
10	99	98

Step 3   The difference in readings for each pair is calculated by subtracting one sample reading from the other. It does not matter which is subtracted from which, as long as you are consistent, but it is easier to subtract in the direction which gives fewest minus signs – in this case subtract the axillary temperature from the mouth temperature. This will give a set of differences which we label 'd'.

Patient	d (mouth temp. minus axillary temp.)	d^2
1	2	4
2	0	0
3	-1	1
4	2	4
5	2	4
6	1	1
7	2	4
8	1	1
9	2	4
10	1	1
	12	24

Now calculate the mean of the d values to get

$$\bar{d} = \frac{12}{10} = 1.2$$

and the standard deviation of the d values to get:

$$S = \sqrt{\frac{\Sigma d^2 - (\Sigma d)^2/n}{n-1}} = \sqrt{\frac{24 - \frac{12^2}{10}}{9}} = 1.03$$

(Note that n = 10, the number of pairs).

The test statistic is

$$t = \frac{\bar{d}}{S/\sqrt{n}} = \frac{1.2}{1.03/\sqrt{10}} = 3.68$$

Step 4   To interpret this result, you use the same t-table as for the one sample test (Table 1, Appendix). Look up the t value for n – 1 degrees of freedom and the 5% level of significance. In this case $t_{9, 5\%} = 2.2622$. The calculated test statistic is greater than this, so the null hypothesis is rejected at the 5% level (with less than a 5% chance of being wrong) and the conclusion is that there is a difference in mouth and underarm temperature.

The advantage of this test is that, because it operates on the difference between paired readings, a good deal of the variability between individuals is removed from the calculations. So the fact that for some individuals both temperatures were relatively high (or low) does not affect the results since we are only using the difference between the readings. This is appropriate because we are not interested in absolute levels of temperature here, but in the relationship between the readings obtained at two sites used in the taking of temperatures.

Two sample independent t-test

The paired t-test considered the mean of two related samples. The two sample independent t-test, as its name suggests, investigates the relationship between the means of two independent samples. As for all t-tests, there is an underlying assumption that the distributions of both samples are Normal with equal standard deviations.

Example You want to know if there is any difference in pulse rates between men and women. Take the pulse rate of a sample of 8 women and a sample of 10 men.

Step 1 The null hypothesis is that there is no difference in the pulse rates of men and women, i.e. your two samples come from the same distribution.

Step 2 Measure the pulse rate of a sample of 8 women and 10 men with the following results.

Pulse rates of women: 70, 73, 72, 72, 71, 74, 75, 72
Pulse rates of men: 72, 72, 70, 74, 76, 74, 72, 72, 73, 71

Step 3 The test statistic is given by

$$t = \frac{\bar{x}_1 - \bar{x}_2}{\sqrt{S^2 \left(\frac{1}{n_1} + \frac{1}{n_2} \right)}}$$

where $\bar{x}_1$ is the mean of the first sample, $\bar{x}_2$ is the mean of the second sample, n_1 is the size of the first sample, n_2 is the size of the second sample; and

$$S^2 = \frac{\Sigma x_1^2 - \frac{(\Sigma x_1)^2}{n_1} + \Sigma x_2^2 - \frac{(\Sigma x_2)^2}{n_2}}{n_1 + n_2 - 2}$$

where Σx_1^2 is the sum of the squares of the first sample, $(\Sigma x_1)^2$ is the sum of the first sample squared, Σx_2^2 is the sum of the squares of the second sample and $(\Sigma x_2)^2$ is the sum of the second sample squared.

(*Hint:* You may calculate all of this on smaller numbers obtained by subtracting any convenient constant from each of the observations.)

Subtracting 70 from every observation gives:

x_1	x_1^2	x_2	x_2^2
0	0	2	4
3	9	2	4
2	4	0	0
2	4	4	16
1	1	6	36
4	16	4	16
5	25	2	4
2	4	2	4
		3	9
		1	1
19	63	26	94

So; $\Sigma x_1 = 19$, $\Sigma x_1^2 = 63$, $\Sigma x_2 = 26$, $\Sigma x_2^2 = 94$, $n_1 = 8$, $n_2 = 10$.

$$S^2 = \frac{63 - \dfrac{19^2}{8} + 94 - \dfrac{26^2}{10}}{8 + 10 - 2} = \frac{17.875 + 26.4}{16} = 2.767$$

$$t = \frac{\dfrac{19}{8} - \dfrac{26}{10}}{\sqrt{2.767 \left(\dfrac{1}{8} + \dfrac{1}{10}\right)}}$$

$$= \frac{2.375 - 2.6}{0.789}$$

$$= -0.285$$

The sign of the t-statistic does not matter so take t as 0.285.

Step 4 Now look up Table 1 in the Appendix to find the tabulated value for t with $(n_1 + n_2 - 2)$ degrees of freedom at the 5% level of significance. In this case $t_{16,5\%} = 2.1199$. The calculated t statistic is smaller than this, so the null hypothesis is accepted and the conclusion is that there is no difference in the pulse rates of men and women. (Had the calculated value been larger than 2.12, you would have rejected the null hypothesis and concluded that there is a difference in the pulse rates of men and women (with a chance of being wrong of less than 5%).)

Two parametric, two sample tests have been described, one for use with related, paired samples and the other for use with independent samples.

Both tests are used with interval level data. Some non-parametric tests will now be described, which can be used with data either at the nominal level of measurement or the ordinal level of measurement.

The McNemar test

This test is particularly applicable to 'before and after' designs in which each person is used as his or her own control. Nominal measurements can be used to assess the 'before to after' change. So this test is for paired readings on subjects in a similar way to its parametric equivalent, the paired t-test.

Example You are interested in the initiation of interaction between learners and trained staff on a ward. You observe the first contact that newly allocated learners make with a member of the trained ward staff on their first day in the ward, and note whether this initial contact is with another learner or with a qualified nurse. You repeat this exercise 30 days into the allocation period. You want to know whether learner to trained staff contacts have increased in number after 30 days.

Step 1 The null hypothesis is that there is no difference in the number of initial contacts between learners and trained staff after 30 days: the number of learner/trained initial contacts on day 1 will not differ significantly from the number of learner/trained initial contacts on day 30.

Step 2 Collect the information with the following results.

Number of learners whose initial contact changed from learner to trained
= 14.
Number of learners whose initial contact changed from trained to learner
= 4.
Number of learners whose initial contact remained another learner = 4.
Number of learners whose initial contact remained a trained nurse = 13.

Put this information in tabular form

| | | 30th day | | | | |
		Trained	Learner			
	Learner	14	4		A	B
1st						
day						
	Trained	13	4		C	D

Calculations are based on the numbers in cells A and D (where changed behaviour occurred). The test statistic is

$$\chi^2 = \frac{(|A - D| - 1)^2}{A + D}$$

where $|A - D|$ is the difference between A and D, ignoring a minus sign if D is bigger than A. So,

$$\chi^2 = \frac{(10 - 1)^2}{18} = \frac{9^2}{18} = \frac{81}{18} = 4.5$$

Step 4 To interpret the results use the chi-squared table (Table 4, Appendix). The figure needed is that for one degree of freedom at the 5% level. So $\chi^2_{1,5\%} = 3,841$. The calculated χ^2 statistic is larger than this, so the null hypothesis is rejected and it is concluded that the number of learner to trained nurse initial contacts after 30 days differs significantly from that on day one (with less than a 5% chance of being wrong).

This is a very useful test which only requires the identification of a change – not the exact measurement of that change. It is therefore suitable when data can only be obtained at the nominal level.

The Wilcoxon signed-ranks test

This is a non-parametric test designed for use with paired readings or ordinal level data.

Ordinal data is required for this test since it takes account not only of the difference in the 'before to after' design, but of the extent of that difference. It is applicable for matched (paired) samples as in a 'before to after' design, like its parametric equivalent the paired t-test.

Example An experimental scheme is to be introduced to improve nurses' communication with patients. A five point scale is devised where scores are allocated as follows during bed-bathing:

    1 = no communication whatever with patient,
    2 = minimal communication on non-threatening topics,
    3 = some communication on how the patient is feeling,
    4 = good communication relating to patient's queries,
    5 = excellent communication on all patient's queries.

It should be noted that further criteria would need to be available to define more exactly the behaviours ascribed to each of the five points of the scale.

This assessment is carried out on ten randomly selected nurses before and after they attend a course on communication. You want to know if the course has been effective in enhancing communication skills.

Step 1 The null hypothesis is that there is no change in communication skills.

Step 2 The assessment is carried out before and after the course with the following results:

Nurse	Before	After
1	3	4
2	2	5
3	3	2
4	4	3
5	1	4
6	5	5
7	4	3
8	5	5
9	2	4
10	2	5

Step 3 The calculation of the test statistic is as follows:

(a) calculate the difference between the 'after' and 'before' scores: 1, 3, −1, −1, 3, 0, −1, 0, 2, 3;

(b) ignoring the positive or negative sign, the differences are ranked after dropping from the analysis any ties (difference of zero).

There are two ties, so these are dropped and we write out in rank order the remaining eight differences, (ignoring the signs): 1, 1, 1, 1, 2, 3, 3, 3.

The first four are all 1, so these share the ranks one to four equally: (1 + 2 + 3 + 4)/4 = 2.5, so each of the first four gets a rank of 2.5. The 2 gets the rank 5, and the three 3s share ranks 6, 7 and 8 to obtain (6 + 7 + 8)/3 = 7, a rank of 7 each. So the ranks are 2.5, 2.5, 2.5, 2.5, 5, 7, 7, 7.

(c) Now attach to each rank the sign of the original difference: 2.5, −2.5, −2.5, −2.5, 5, 7, 7, 7.

(d) Now add up the positive ranks and the negative ranks.

sum of positive ranks =	2.5	sum of negative ranks =	−2.5
	5.0		−2.5
	7.0		−2.5
	7.0		
	7.0		
	———		———
	28.5		−7.5

The test-statistic T is the smaller sum (ignoring the sign), so T = 7.5.

Step 4 To interpret this result, use Table 5 in the Appendix. Look up the tabulated figure for the appropriate degrees of freedom (equal to the effective sample size after ties are dropped) and the 5% significance level. In this case $T_{8,5\%}$ = 3. The figure of 7.5 you have calculated is greater than the tabulated T, so *accept* the null hypothesis and conclude that the course makes no difference to communication skills. (Note that this is the first test where a calculated test statistic greater than the tabulated values means that you accept the null hypothesis.)

Having looked at two non-parametric tests for two related samples, a non-parametric test for two independent samples will finally be considered.

The Mann–Whitney U test
This is a non-parametric test for two independent samples, and is the non-parametric equivalent of the two sample, independent t-test. It is best used on data where the assumptions for the t-test are not met, or where the level of measurement is weaker than interval level.

Example　A test schedule has been devised which measures management potential in newly qualified staff nurses. This schedule is scored by adding up ticked items observed during the normal ward routine. The total score represents the number of ticked items out of 120. The question is whether there is any difference in the management potential of graduate nurses and nurses trained in traditional schools of nursing.

Step 1　The null hypothesis is that there is no difference in management potential between recently qualified graduate and recently qualified non-graduate staff nurses.

Step 2　The test schedules are carried out on a random sample of four graduate and five non-graduate staff nurses in a large ward of a hospital with the following results

Graduates (G)	Non-graduates (N)
110	78
70	64
53	75
51	45
	82

Step 3　The calculation of the test statistic is as follows.

(a)　arrange the scores in order of size, retaining the identity of each:

45	51	53	64	70	75	78	82	110
N	G	G	N	G	N	N	N	G

(b)　Calculate the test statistic, U, by counting the total number of N scores preceding each G score: $1 + 1 + 2 + 5 = 9$

Step 4　To interpret the results, use Table 6 in the Appendix. The degrees of freedom are given by the two sample sizes. The critical value is found by searching for the value in the table corresponding to $n_1 = 4$ and $n_2 = 5$. This value is 1. Since the calculated U value is greater than 1, the null hypothesis is accepted and the conclusion is that there is no difference in management potential between graduate and non-graduate staff nurses.

The χ^2 (chi-squared) two sample test
This test is a non-parametric test which explores the relationship between

two independent variables by looking at the distribution among categories of the two variables, and comparing this with the distribution which would be expected under a null hypothesis that the two variables are independent. The detail of the calculation of this test is given in the next chapter, which is devoted to relationships between two variables. The chi-squared test should be noted in this chapter, however, as a non-parametric method for two samples of data which can be applied to ordinal level data.

Summary

The previous chapter concentrated on ways to describe a variable. This chapter goes a step further in dealing with a series of hypotheses about one or two variables, which can be tested and the inferences which can be made from such tests.

In dealing with your own data, the first step is to write down concisely the hypothesis which you wish to test. Then answer the following questions.

1. Do I need a one sample or two sample test?
2. Is the data measured at ordinal, nominal or interval level?
3. Do I know that the underlying distribution of my variable or variables is Normal? If not, is it symmetrical, bell-shaped and continuous in which case I could use a parametric test. If not, I need a non-parametric test.

Then use the table of tests earlier in this chapter (page 76) to identify a group of possible tests and choose the one which allows your particular hypothesis to be tested.

There are many more statistical tests than those described in this chapter. Once you have mastered the four steps, you should be able to consult any standard basic statistical test book and carry out other tests, not covered here. In this way you will get the most out of the data you have collected and you will obtain the maximum benefit from the use of statistical inference.

6

Association, Correlation and Regression

Caution in interpretation

This chapter is devoted to the relationship between variables. When two variables are related in some way, there is association or correlation between them. For example, men are associated with beer drinking. We mean by this that a greater proportion of men than of women tend to drink beer. So the association of men and beer drinking means that men rather than women tend to drink beer. But many women also drink beer.

Perhaps the best known association is that of smoking and lung cancer. A greater proportion of smokers than of non-smokers get lung cancer. But non-smokers also get lung cancer, albeit in vastly smaller proportions than smokers. Many people say that smoking *causes* lung cancer. We ourselves believe that smoking is *a cause of* lung cancer on the basis of the evidence from laboratory experiments that the persistent action of cigarette smoke on cells will cause cell degeneration which can lead to cells becoming cancerous. It is important to recognise, however, that the existence of association does not itself automatically prove cause and effect. This is the most common misinterpretation of statistical procedures such as the measurement of association or correlation.

Proving cause and effect is the concern of many health researchers. This is understandable, because once the cause of a disease is known, it may be possible to find a means of preventing it. But nothing is more difficult to prove than cause and effect. This is because there is rarely one single cause for any effect. A multiplicity of factors probably come into play, and, in health research, it is often impossible to separate out these factors.

Coronary heart disease provides a good illustration of the difficulties. What causes coronary heart disease? There is some evidence to support the hypothesis that fat in dietary intake is a factor, smoking is thought to be a factor, stress is recognised by many to be a factor, as, no doubt, is socio-economic status which is correlated with most diseases. How can we unravel all of this? You could probably establish association of each of the factors cited with coronary heart disease. Yet there are no doubt people who smoke, eat fatty foods and suffer from high levels of stress and deprivation who will not get coronary heart disease. All that can be done is take account of the weight of evidence while recognising that it is unlikely that incontrovertible proof of cause and effect can ever be established.

There is a second reason for caution in interpreting an association or correlation. It is possible that an apparently strong association or correlation is quite spurious. For example, any two factors which both increase over time could be measured to show a positive correlation. For instance, the sales of television sets and the incidence of schizophrenia in the post-war decades would appear to be highly correlated, when in reality there is unlikely to be any direct relationship whatever. Likewise a positive correlation would probably be found between ice-cream sales and the numbers of over 70-year-old people in hospital beds in the last decade. But you would not conclude that there was any connection between ice-cream consumption and the demand for geriatric care, still less that ice-cream caused the increased demand! Common sense is the best preventative measure for dealing with spurious association! But it is not always easy to detect when a measured correlation supports ones intuition.

Exploration of the relationship between two variables begins by looking first at ways to establish the existence of association. The next step is to calculate measures of association and the strength and direction of correlation. Finally the value of one variable is predicted from another.

The existence of association

The existence of a relationship between two variables can be explored if we have data even at the nominal level of measurement. Nominal level measurement exists when we know how many subjects fall into the various categories of each of the two variables.

Chi-squared test

This test can be used to see if there is a relationship between two variables following the drawing up of a contingency table.

Example 1   Say that we want to know if there is any association between the sector of nursing and gender of the nurse. (The membership of the sectors should be exclusive: it should not be possible for an individual subject to belong to more than one category.) Are there more male nurses in education or administration than in hospital or community based nursing?

We collect information on 200 nurses, 60 in hospital, 40 in community nursing, 50 in education and 50 in administration. We can now draw up the contingency table.

	Male	Female	Total
Hospital	15	45	60
Community	5	35	40
Education	25	25	50
Administration	35	15	50
Total	80	120	200

The *row total* for hospital is 60, for community is 40, for education is 50 and for administration is 50. The *column total* for males is 80 and for females is 120. The *grand total* is 200.

A test can now be carried out to determine if there is an association between gender and sector. The usual four steps in a significance test are used.

Step 1   The null hypothesis is that there is no association between gender of the nurse and sector of nursing.

Step 2   The data were collected and the results tabulated as shown above in the contingency table.

Step 3   The calculation of the test statistic is as follows.

(a) Calculate an expected value (to reflect the assumption that the proportion of males and females is the same for each sector) for each cell of the contingency table if the null hypothesis were true. For each cell, the expected value, E, is given by:

$$E = \frac{\text{row total} \times \text{column total}}{\text{grand total}}$$

So for the hospital/male cell (observed value, O = 15)

$$E = \frac{60 \times 80}{200} = 24$$

For the education/female cell (observed value, O = 25)

$$E = \frac{50 \times 120}{200} = 30$$

Repeating the calculation of the expected value for each cell will give the following table of *expected* values:

	Male	Female	Total
Hospital	24	36	60
Community	16	24	40
Education	20	30	50
Administration	20	30	50
Total	80	120	200

Note that the row and column totals and the grand total of the expected values should equal those in the table of observed values. This is always a good check on the arithmetic.

(b) Now calculate the test statistic $\chi^2 = \Sigma \dfrac{(O - E)^2}{E}$

		O	E	O – E	$(O - E)^2$	$(O - E)^2/E$
Hospital	M	15	24	–9	81	3.375
	F	45	36	9	81	2.25
Community	M	5	16	–11	121	7.563
	F	35	24	11	121	5.042
Education	M	25	20	5	25	1.25
	F	25	30	–5	25	0.833
Administration	M	35	20	15	225	11.25
	F	15	30	–15	225	7.5
						39.063

So $\chi^2 = \Sigma \dfrac{(O - E)^2}{E} = 39.063$

Step 4 Interpret the result by looking up the tabulated value of χ^2 with $[(r - 1) \times (c - 1)]$ degrees of freedom, where r is the number of rows in the contingency table and c is the number of columns. In this case r = 4 and c = 2, so $[(r - 1) \times (c - 1)] = 3 \times 1 = 3$, so we want the χ^2 figure with 3 degrees of freedom at the 5% level, i.e. $\chi^2 = 7.815$ (see Table 4, Appendix). Our calculated χ^2 is larger than this so we reject the null hypothesis at the 5% level (with a less than 5% chance of being wrong) and conclude that there is an association between gender of the nurse and sector of nursing.

A χ^2 test of association can be applied to two variables with any number of categories, using the above method. (The only exception is the 2×2 contingency table which is covered in the next section.)

Example 2 The following contingency table gives the breakdown of grade by age for enrolled nurses and staff nurses in a 3×2 contingency table.

Age	Staff Nurse	SEN	Total
Less than 22	10	5	15
22–23.9	50	15	65
Over 24	30	40	70
Total	90	60	150

Step 1 The null hypothesis is that there is no association between age and grade of nurse.

Step 2 Collect data as above.

Step 3 As in the previous example, calculate the expected numbers in each cell (E = (row total × column total)/grand total), for example

$$E = \frac{15 \times 90}{150} = 9$$

Then carry out the calculation as before.

Observed (O)	Expected (E)	O − E	$(O - E)^2$	$(O - E)^2/E$
10	9	1	1	0.111
5	6	−1	1	0.167
50	39	11	121	3.103
15	26	−11	121	4.654
30	42	−12	144	3.429
40	28	12	144	5.143
				16.607

$$\chi^2 = \Sigma \frac{(O - E)^2}{E} = 16.607$$

Step 4 Compare with tabulated χ^2 with $[(r - 1) \times (c - 1)]$ degrees of freedom; r = 3, c = 2, so (r − 1) × (c − 1) = 2 × 1 = 2. So we need $\chi^2_{2,5\%}$ = 5.991. The calculated test statistic is larger so we reject the null hypothesis at the 5% level (with a chance of less than 5% of being wrong) and conclude that there is an association between age and grade of nurse.

Uses and limitations of the χ^2 test
The χ^2 test has been illustrated with a 4 × 2 contingency and a 3 × 2 contingency table. Apart from the 2 × 2 table which is a special case, any dimensions can be handled using the same method – 7 × 4 or 16 × 13 or whatever. Just remember to adjust the degrees of freedom in Step 4 of the significance test.

Finally, there is one very important caveat in carrying out χ^2 tests as described. The test becomes invalid and must not be used if

(a) any cell has an expected frequency of less than one, *or*
(b) more than 20% of the cells have an expected frequency of less than five.

If either (a) or (b) holds, when you have calculated your expected values, *do not proceed with the test*. There are two things you can do.

1. Combine adjacent categories to increase the expected frequencies if it is sensible to do so and then proceed with the test on the new contingency table. You could, for instance, sensibly combine age categories (in the 3 × 2 example you could combine 'less than 22' and '22–23.9' to give a category 'less than 24'), but you could not sensibly combine apples and oranges! In general, you can normally combine categories of ordinal variables but not nominal variables.
2. If you cannot combine categories, carry out some alternative test as

discussed in, for example Siegel (1956). The χ^2 should not be used in these circumstances.

The χ^2 2 × 2 test

A special case of the χ^2 test is for a 2 × 2 contingency table. The following method should only be used if the grand total is at least 20 and no expected frequency is less than five. If either of these conditions are not met an alternative test should be used (see Fisher's Exact Probability Test, Siegel (1956)).

Example You want to know whether there is an association between pass rate in final examinations and type of training (register or roll). This question actually arose in considering manpower needs and their implications for nurse training.

Step 1 The null hypothesis is that there is no association between pass rates and type of training undertaken.

Step 2 Data on examination performance are collected on a sample of 40 students and 60 pupils with the following results

	Pass	Fail	Total
Students	35	5	40
Pupils	52	8	60
Total	87	13	100

In general the 2 × 2 contingency table may be represented

a	b	D
c	d	C
A	B	N

Step 3 The test statistic is calculated as follows:

$$\chi^2 = \frac{N\left[\,|ad - bc| \, - \, \dfrac{N}{2}\right]^2}{ABCD}$$

$$= \frac{100[\,|(35 \times 8) - (5 \times 52)| - 50]^2}{87 \times 13 \times 40 \times 60}$$

$$= \frac{100[(280 - 260) - 50]^2}{2714400}$$

$$= \frac{100(20 - 50)^2}{2714400}$$

$$= \frac{100 \times 900}{2714400}$$

$$= 0.033$$

N.B. Had |ad – bc| been a negative number (if bc was greater than ad), you simply reverse the sign and take it as the positive value.

Step 4   Look up the tabulated χ^2 with one degree of freedom at the 5% level which is $\chi^2 = 3.841$ (Table 4, Appendix). Since the calculated χ^2 is less than this value, we accept the null hypothesis that there is no association between pass rates and type of training.

The various ways in which a χ^2 test can assist in establishing whether there is an association or relationship between two variables have now been covered. We will now go a step further and show how to represent graphically and measure the strength and direction of the relationship. This is the realm of correlation analysis.

The strength and direction of a relationship: correlation

Although the terms 'association' and 'correlation' are used fairly interchangeably, one distinction in practice is that correlation is more often applied to interval level data. Measures of association, like the χ^2 test, can be applied to nominal data. With interval level data on two variables, a helpful first step is to plot the data on a scattergram.

Scattergram

Example   You want to know if test scores on practical assessments are related to written examination performance. For a random sample of 10 students, the scores on practical and written performance were as follows.

Student	Practical assessment mark (out of total of 20)	Written examination mark (out of a total of 40)
1	15	27
2	6	10
3	14	28
4	10	16
5	9	20
6	11	19
7	14	26
8	13	26
9	8	15
10	5	8

These marks can be represented as a scattergram, such as Fig. 6.1. Inspection of this graph reveals that there does appear to be a relationship between the two sets of marks. As the practical assessment mark goes up, the written examination mark goes up, and the relationship looks fairly linear since you

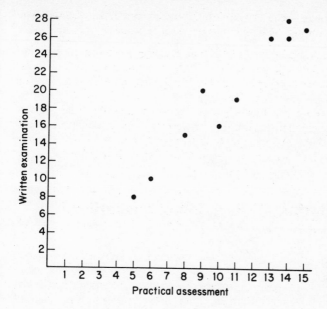

Fig. 6.1 Scattergram.

could draw a reasonably straight line through the points without any point being too far from the line.

The drawing of a scattergram is a useful first step since it will allow you to make a visual assessment of the direction and strength and nature of any correlation which might be present. A series of scattergrams is provided here and guidance given on how to interpret them in terms of correlation. In each case we are looking at a scattergram of two variables x and y, plotted from low to high on their respective axes.

Positive linear patterns These are observed when y goes from low to high as x goes from low to high. If you imagine a line drawn through the points it will rise from left to right.

Scattergrams (a)–(c) in Fig. 6.2 show some evidence of positive correlation. In (a), the points lies on a perfect straight line indicating a strong relationship between x and y. In (b) there is a clear trend towards a positive correlation, although by no means all of the points will lie on a straight line. This indicates a moderate positive relationship. In (c) there is a very slight trend suggesting positive correlation, but if a line were drawn through the points, many points would lie far off the line. This indicates a weak positive relationship.

Negative linear patterns These are observed when y goes from high to low as x goes from low to high. If you imagine a line drawn through the points it

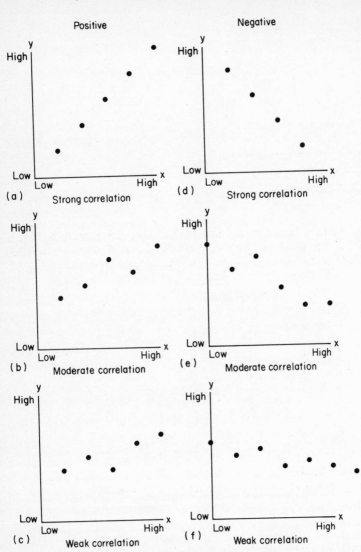

Fig. 6.2 Positive (a, b, c) and negative (d, e, f) correlations.

will fall from left to right, illustrated by Fig. 6.2 (d), (e) and (f). These three scattergrams indicate strong, moderate and weak negative correlation respectively.

Other patterns   If no correction, either positive or negative is present, the scattergram would look something like Fig. 6.3.

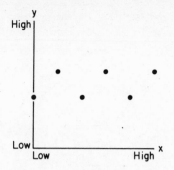

Fig. 6.3 No correlation.

So far we have looked only at linear correlation. It is possible to have a curvilinear correlation and, although the calculation of correlation will not be covered in this instance, Fig. 6.4 provides helpful illustrations of it.

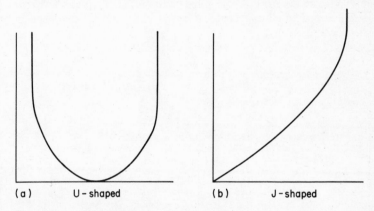

Fig. 6.4 Curvilinear patterns.

It should be clear that one benefit of first drawing a scattergram is that you can then see if the correlation is linear or curvilinear. If it looks linear, we can proceed to measure it.

Correlation coefficients

The two measures of correlation (sometimes called correlation coefficients) described here are standardised to take values ranging from -1 to $+1$. These values may be broadly interpreted as follows.

Maximum negative correlation				Maximum positive correlation
-1	-0.5	0	$+0.5$	$+1$
	Moderate negative correlation	No correlation	Moderate positive correlation	

So Fig. 6.2 (a) would have a score of 1, (b) would score between 0.4 and 0.6, and (c) would score about 0.05 or 0.1. Figure 6.2 (d) would have a score of -1, (e) between -0.4 and -0.6 and (f) around -0.05 or -0.1 on the negative side. Figure 6.3 would score a small positive or negative close to zero. The detail of the calculation of two correlation coefficients is described below.

The product moment correlation coefficient (Pearson, 1924)
For this calculation, interval level data is needed.

Example   We can use the example given earlier in this chapter on written and practical examinations. For two variables x and y, the Pearson coefficient, r, is given by:

$$ r = \frac{\Sigma xy - \dfrac{\Sigma x \Sigma y}{n}}{\sqrt{\Sigma x^2 - \dfrac{(\Sigma x)^2}{n}}\ \sqrt{\Sigma y^2 - \dfrac{(\Sigma y)^2}{n}}} $$

To calculate this carry out the following procedures:

x (practical) assessment	x^2	y (written) examination	y^2	xy
15	225	27	729	405
6	36	10	100	60
14	196	28	784	392
10	100	16	256	160
9	81	20	400	180
11	121	19	361	209
14	196	26	676	364
13	169	26	676	338
8	64	15	225	120
5	25	8	64	40
105	1213	195	4271	2268

The final column is obtained by multiplying each x by its y partner. Substitute these figures, with n = 10, in the above equation.

$$r = \frac{2268 - \dfrac{105 \times 195}{10}}{\sqrt{1213 - \dfrac{105^2}{10}} \; \sqrt{4271 - \dfrac{195^2}{10}}}$$

$$= \frac{2268 - 2047.5}{\sqrt{1213 - 1102.5} \; \sqrt{4271 - 3802.5}}$$

$$= \frac{220.5}{\sqrt{110.5} \; \sqrt{468.5}}$$

$$= \frac{220.5}{10.5 \times 21.64} = \frac{220.5}{227.2} = 0.97$$

So as expected from the scattergram we have a strong positive correlation of $+0.97$. Had our r value been smaller, however, the question could have arisen as to how to establish whether the level of correlation present is significant or not. We will illustrate a hypothesis test using the above result. Note that this significance test requires the assumption of a normal distribution.

Step 1 The null hypothesis is that there is no correlation between the practical assessment and written examination results.

Step 2 The data is as above.

Step 3 The test statistic is

$$t = \frac{r\sqrt{N-2}}{\sqrt{1-r^2}}$$

$$= \frac{0.97\sqrt{8}}{\sqrt{1 - 0.97^2}}$$

$$= \frac{0.97 \times 2.828}{\sqrt{1 - 0.941}} = \frac{2.743}{\sqrt{0.059}} = \frac{2.743}{0.243} = 11.288$$

where N is the number of pairs of observation.

Step 4 To interpret this result compare it with a tabulated t value with $N - 2$ degrees of freedom at the 5% level (Table 1, Appendix). The value for $t_{8,5\%}$ is 2.306. Our calculated value is large so we can reject the NH at the 5% level (with less than a 5% chance of error) and conclude that there is significant correlation between written and practical examination performance.

The Spearman rank correlation coefficient
This coefficient of correlation can be calculated using interval or ordinal data. No distributional assumptions about the data are required in testing the significance of the correlation.

Example   Two ward sisters meet to discuss the reports on a batch of learners whose allocation is just ending. They decide to rank the twelve learners in order of clinical ability, independently of each other. The question arises as to how consistent the two sets of ranks are: is Sister A's ranking correlated with that of Sister B? The ranks given were as follows.

Student	Rank given by Sister A	Rank given by Sister B
A	2	3
B	6	4
C	5	2
D	1	1
E	10	8
F	9	11
G	8	10
H	3	6
I	4	7
J	12	12
K	7	5
L	11	9

With ranked data, the Spearman rank correlation coefficient, r_s, may be calculated. It is given by

$$r_s = 1 - \frac{6\Sigma d^2}{N^3 - N}$$

where d is the difference in rank (Sister A − Sister B) and N is the number of pairs of observations. In this case the differences are

Student	Difference in rank, d	d^2
A	−1	1
B	2	4
C	3	9
D	0	0
E	2	4
F	−2	4
G	−2	4
H	−3	9
I	−3	9
J	0	0
K	2	4
L	2	4
		Σd^2 = 52

So, $r_s = 1 - \dfrac{6 \times 52}{12^3 - 12}$

$$= 1 - \frac{312}{1728 - 12}$$

$$= 1 - \frac{312}{1716}$$

$$= 1 - 0.18$$

$$= 0.82$$

The value of the Spearman rank correlation coefficient confirms that there is a strong positive correlation with a value of $+0.82$. To test whether this is a significant correlation:

Step 1 The null hypothesis is that there is no correlation in the two sets of scores.

Step 2 Collect data as above.

Step 3 Calculate $r_s = 0.82$ as above.

Step 4 Find the tabulated value for $N = 12$ at the 5% level. (Table 7, Appendix). This is 0.5874. Our calculated value is greater than this so we can reject the NH at the 5% level and conclude that there is significant correlation between the rankings of the two sisters.

Association between variables, and the strength and direction of correlation between variables have now been established. The final step is to use one variable to predict another. This technique is called regression.

Regression analysis

Consider again the scattergram of the practical marks against the written marks of ten learners (page 97). We noted that there appeared to be a strong positive linear relationship, and we proceeded to confirm that there was a correlation of 0.97. Regression analysis is the technique which enables us to find the best straight line through the points. Once we have found this line we can use it to predict one variable from the other.

But what is the 'best' straight line. You could, for example, join the first and last points together to obtain a straight line. Or you could join the first and the penultimate point to obtain a slightly different straight line. There are, in fact, an infinite number of straight lines which could be drawn through this set of points.

Whichever line you draw, not all points will fall on the line. Think of the vertical distance from each point to the line as the error associated with that point (Fig. 6.5).

The regression technique called 'least squares' finds the line with the minimum total squared error.

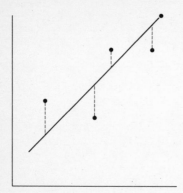

Fig. 6.5 The error in drawing a straight line through a set of points.

To find this line, we need only apply two simple formulae. Any straight line can be written y = a + bx where a is the intercept on the y axis, and b is the slope of the line (Fig. 6.6). The 'best' line using least squares regression is given by the formula y = a + bx, where y = written examination mark, x = practical assessment mark,

$$b = \frac{\Sigma xy - \dfrac{\Sigma x \Sigma y}{n}}{\Sigma x^2 - \dfrac{(\Sigma x)^2}{n}}$$

and a = $\bar{y}$ − b$\bar{x}$.

For the data on written and practical examinations, we have already calculated most of the parts of these formulae (in doing the Pearson correlation coefficient, page 100).

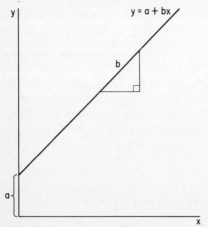

Fig. 6.6 The graph of a straight line.

So, $b = \dfrac{2268 - \dfrac{105 \times 195}{10}}{1213 - \dfrac{105^2}{10}} = \dfrac{220.5}{110.5} = 2.00$

and $a = \dfrac{195}{10} - \left(2.00 \times \dfrac{105}{10}\right)$

$= 19.5 - (2.00 \times 10.5)$

$= 19.5 - 21$

$= -1.5$

So the equation of the regression line is

y (written exam mark) $= -1.5 + 2.00x$ (practical exam mark)

For every value of x we already have an observed y value. But we can now predict the y value for each value of x using this formula. For example the observed x of 15 was associated with an observed y of 27. The predicted y from the regression line is $-1.5 + (2.00 \times 15) = 28.5$.

In this way we can now look at a table of observed and predicted y values

x	Observed y	Predicted $y = -1.5 + 2.00x$
15	27	28.5
6	10	10.5
14	28	26.5
10	16	18.5
9	20	16.5
11	19	20.5
14	26	26.5
13	26	24.5
8	15	14.5
5	8	8.5

You can see that the observed and predicted values are very close and while no point lies exactly on the line, all are very close to it. In this case we have a good linear fit.

If these results were real, you might now want to ask if there is any point in doing both written and practical examinations since you can make a good prediction of the written mark from the practical mark. Although this is true, in the professional fields in particular it is valuable to use a number of different types of assessment.

One advantage is that you can now predict written marks from new values of practical marks, provided they lie within the range of the data. For example, say another student obtained 12 in the practical examination but was ill and missed the written test. You can now predict that her written mark would be about

$-1.5 + (2.00 \times 12) = 22.5.$

Note that no value of 12 appeared in the original set of marks but you can now predict from it since it lies within the range of marks considered.

You could reverse the above example and predict practical marks from written marks. In this case the formula for the regression line is

$$x = a^\star + b^\star y$$

where $a^\star$ is the intercept of the line (and we denote it by $a^\star$ to distinguish from a, the intercept of the line predicting y from x, which has just been calculated), and $b^\star$ is the slope of the line (and we denote it by $b^\star$ to distinguish from b, the slope of the line predicting y from x, which has just been calculated).

$$b^\star = \frac{\Sigma xy - \dfrac{\Sigma x \Sigma y}{n}}{\Sigma y^2 - \dfrac{(\Sigma y)^2}{n}}$$

(Note that due to regression this way round, the bottom line of the formula changes.)

and $a^\star = \bar{x} - b^\star \bar{y}$

Using the calculations already performed for the Pearson correlation coefficient:

$$\Sigma xy = 2268, \Sigma x = 105, \Sigma y = 195, \Sigma y^2 = 4271, n = 10$$

So, $b^\star = \dfrac{2268 - \dfrac{105 \times 195}{10}}{4271 - \dfrac{195^2}{10}} = \dfrac{220.5}{468.5} = 0.47$

and $a^\star = 10.5 - (0.47 \times 19.5)$
$= 1.34$

So, x (practical exam mark) $= 1.34 + 0.47y$ (written mark)

We can now draw up a table of observed x values, observed y values and predicted x values.

x (observed)	x (predicted) x = 1.34 + 0.47 y	y (observed)
15	14.0	27
6	6.0	10
14	14.5	28
10	8.9	16
9	10.7	20
11	10.3	19
14	13.6	26
13	13.6	26
8	8.4	15
5	5.1	8

Again you can see that the regression line is a good predictor of the observed values. If you had a student who sat the written examination and was awarded a score of 22, you could use this regression line to predict her practical score if she missed this examination.

$$x \text{ (practical exam mark)} = 1.34 + 0.47 \, y \text{ (written mark)}$$
$$= 1.34 + (0.47 \times 22)$$
$$= 11.68$$

So regression can be carried out on either variable, but it is important to remember the change of formula if you want to regress on the other variable.

Summary

This chapter has covered a range of techniques for investigating the relationship between variables. Carrying out these techniques is the easy part! The difficult stage in this area is in interpreting the meaning of significant results. The important thing is not to overclaim – if you have found an association, resist the temptation to say it is cause and effect. By all means say that the results showing strong associations or correlations suggest a causative relationship, but stop there. And be very suspicious of anyone else who *claims* cause and effect on the basis of the techniques included in this chapter!

7

Research and Nursing Practice

We began this book by asserting that research should be a routine part of the nurse's working skills. Having in later chapters gone through the stages of the research process, it may well seem to the reader that the scale and complexity of research are such that it cannot be accommodated within an already busy working day. In practice, however, only parts of the process we described in Chapters 2 and 3 will be relevant to any particular research problem. To illustrate that research can be a practically feasible, relevant and useful aid, we will end by describing three small, hypothetical pieces of research, one in nurse education, one in nurse management and one in clinical practice.

A small research project in nursing education

A school of nursing was becoming concerned about its recruitment of student nurses. The numbers of applicants had been dropping and tutors who lived in the local community believed that fears of being unemployed when qualified were discouraging potential applicants. There was local talk of nurses training to join the dole queues and that nurse training was a 'waste' of three years. The tutors themselves were not sure to what extent this was true. They decided therefore to carry out a postal survey to investigate the experiences of newly qualified nurses in seeking employment.

A nurse tutor had kept in touch with previous students through producing a newsletter, so she had a full set of current addresses. From these a cohort was chosen of 60 nurses who had qualified 18 months previously. A brief questionnaire was designed by the tutors.

QUESTIONNAIRE

Employment history since qualification   Code _____

1. (a) Please list all nursing posts for which you have applied since you qualified, indicating in each case whether you were interviewed and whether you were successful or not. In the second column place a tick if you were interviewed and a cross if you were not. In the third column place a tick if you were successful and a cross if you were not.

Post applied for (please state grade of post and institution)	**Interviewed?** (please tick for 'yes' and cross for 'no')	**Successful?** (please tick for 'yes' and cross for 'no')
Example: Staff Nurse, Western Hospital	✔	✗

   (b) Please asterisk your current post (if any) in the above table, in the left hand margin.

2. (a) Please list any non-nursing posts for which you have applied since you qualified, indicating in each case whether you were interviewed and whether you were successful.

Posts applied for (please state grade of post and institution)	**Interviewed?** (please tick for 'yes' and cross for 'no')	**Successful?** (please tick for 'yes' and cross for 'no')

   (b) Please asterisk your current post (if any) in the above table, in the left hand margin.

3. If you have not applied for any nursing post since you qualified, please state the reasons.

    _____

    _____

    _____

4. If you have not applied for any post, nursing or non-nursing, since you qualified please state the reasons.

    _____

    _____

    _____

5. If you are currently not working, is this because (please tick)

    (i) not seeking work for family or other personal reasons _____

    (ii) not able to find work _____

    (iii) other – please state reason _____

    _____

    _____

    _____

This questionnaire was piloted on a group of enrolled nurses who were in the school of nursing for an in-service study day. The pilot study confirmed that there was no ambiguity in the questions and that there was enough space in the tables to allow all posts applied for to be included.

The questionnaire was sent out to the 60 nurses, with a pre-paid return envelope and a covering letter explaining the purpose of the study. The letter read as shown opposite.

Before dispatch, each questionnaire was given a code number and a master list of names and codes was kept in a secure place by one senior tutor. As questionnaires were returned, names were deleted from the list. After three weeks, 25 replies had been received and no more had come in for a week. At this point a second copy of the questionnaire and the covering letter and pre-paid return envelope were sent out to the 35 people who had not replied. A further 15 replies came in during the next fortnight. A week later a final posting was sent to the remaining 20 non-respondents and 10 more replies were received over a three week period. At this point a total of 50 replies had been received. This provided a very acceptable response rate of $50/60 \times 100 = 83\%$.

Dear   ,
We are concerned about the employment experiences of the nurses who trained in our School of Nursing. We are sending this questionnaire to everyone who qualified in February 1985 and are asking for some brief information on their experiences since then. We hope that the survey will demonstrate that most of our qualifiers have found employment, and that by publicising this we can reassure the public that nursing is a career with good employment prospects. We have been rather worried about falling applications to the school recently.

Your reply will be treated in absolute confidence and your name will not appear on any record kept of this study. You will notice a code on the questionnaire. This is so that we can keep a check on returned questionnaires and send out follow-up questionnaires to those who do not respond. Once the survey information is received, we will destroy our list of names and codes and the results will be presented anonymously.

I hope that you will help us by returning your questionnaire as soon as possible. Thank you for your co-operation.

Yours sincerely,

Miss E Jones,
Director of Nurse Education

The analysis was performed by a group of tutors who set aside three afternoons to work together on the findings. A number of questions were formulated, to which answers from the data were then sought.

Question: How many jobs in total did the fifty respondents apply for?

Answer: A total of 100 jobs were applied for; on average two per respondent.

Question: How many had found a job since qualifying? How many were in current employment? Why were those currently unemployed not working?

Answer: Forty-five had found a job since qualifying, and of those 40 were in current employment, 37 in nursing posts and three in other posts. Of the ten not currently employed, one was seeking employment as a nurse and three were seeking other employment. Five were not seeking employment for family or other personal reasons and one was undertaking a degree course in nursing.

Question: How many posts had the respondents held since qualifying?

Answer: Thirty had held one post, nine had held two posts and six had held three or more posts. A total of 70 posts had been held by the 50 respondents.

Question: How many respondents had applied for non-nursing posts? What kind of non-nursing posts were applied for?

Answer: Six respondents had applied for non-nursing posts of which two had found posts as unqualified social workers, one as a clerk and three were still unemployed.

A brief summary of these findings was then produced in tabular form.

Currently in nursing posts	37
Currently in non-nursing posts	3
Still seeking employment as nurses	1
Still seeking employment not in nursing	3
Not seeking employment (family and other personal reasons)	5
Further study	1
	50

The results confirmed that the vast majority of those who sought nursing posts were successful, although many had had to apply for more than one post before obtaining a post. A press release was issued, drawing attention to this conclusion, which it was hoped would reassure the public about employment prospects in nursing.

A small research project in nurse management

A senior nursing officer became concerned when she learned that there were plans to close a school of nursing, School A, some 30 miles away and to divert learners to another school some 50 miles away, School B. She felt that this might seriously affect recruitment of qualified staff, since her impression was that many of the staff in her hospital trained at School A.

She decided to do a small study on the present hospital staff to find out where they had trained. Realising that this was a question on the application forms, which were retained in the personnel record of successful applicants, she requested permission to extract this information from the records of all qualified nurses in the hospital.

She designed a form on which to collect the information. A separate form was used for enrolled and registered nurses.

Form used to record information

Training school	
School A	
School B	
Other schools	

As each record was checked, a tick was placed against School A or School B. Where another school had been attended, the name of the school was added under 'Other schools'.

The results were

Registered Nurses		Enrolled Nurses	
School	Number trained	School	Number trained
School A	75	School A	55
School B	60	School B	20
School C	30	School D	15
School E	10	School E	5
Other schools	5	Other schools	5
	Total 180		Total 100

The findings on registered nurses indicated that four schools had produced most of the qualified staff and that School A and School B had both provided substantial numbers of staff. There was no evidence to suggest that the hospital was not attractive to applicants who trained in School B.

The picture for enrolled nurses looked rather different. Over half of them had trained in School A compared to only 20% in School B. There would be some concern about future recruitment of enrolled nurses if School A were closed.

While this small study was not definitive, it represented a systematic effort in gathering relevant information. It could not prove that the closure of School A would have a detrimental effect on recruitment, but it did suggest that there could be problems in recruiting enrolled nurses. This information would be likely to be helpful in support of the case against closure.

A small research project in clinical practice

A sister working on a male surgical ward had been reading about the management of pain (McCaffrey, 1979). She began to wonder how effective was the care of the patients in her ward in relation to the management of pain. She decided to adapt an already published pain assessment scale to examine the post-operative pain experienced by her patients. She prepared the scale used in large black print on a white card as shown below

Excruciating	5
Very Severe	4
Severe	3
Moderate	2
Just noticeable	1
No pain	0

Please indicate how much pain you have at the moment.

The ward was a very busy one and this had to be taken into account when deciding on how many patients to include and how often and when she would assess their level of pain. The population was all the patients undergoing surgery and she decided to take a sample of these and had to decide how to select this sample.

In order to reduce the number of variables involved she decided to include only those undergoing major abdominal surgery, excluding such operations as appendicectomy or herniorrhaphy. She also wanted to have a random sample of patients, if possible but eventually decided to include the first 10 patients undergoing major abdominal surgery in a designated week. She could not think of any reason why there should be any systematic bias in the order in which the patients underwent surgery and considered that this was as random as could be achieved in the circumstances.

One of the staff nurses was also interested in the subject and between them they decided that it was feasible to ask patients to identify their level of pain four times a day for the first two days post-operatively.

At this stage she decided to talk to the consultant and the nursing officer, both of whom thought this was a useful idea. As it was a clear development in nursing assessment they did not think that formal ethical approval was needed.

A sheet to record the results was drawn up and all the scores were added up to give a total score. The maximum possible score for each patient over the two days was 40.

Result recording sheet

Patient	Operation	Age	Day 1				Day 2				Total
			9am	1pm	5pm	9pm	9am	1pm	5pm	9pm	
A											
B											
C											
D											
E											
F											
G											
H											
I											
J											

The results obtained were as follows.

Patient	Total score
A	19
B	18
C	20
D	10
E	17
F	12
G	22
H	14
I	14
J	15
	161

This gives a mean of 16.1 per patient, with an average score of 2.01 on each occasion measured. This indicates an average level of a 'moderate' degree of pain experienced. These results were discussed by all staff on the ward and it was generally agreed that patients should not suffer so much pain after an operation. They decided that they would all read some of the literature on pain and its management (which could be obtained from the School of Nursing and/or Postgraduate Medical Centre Libraries) and then discuss what they had found out and how they might use this knowledge in their practice. It was also felt that it would be useful to invite the houseman working on the ward to join them in this exercise.

During the next four weeks all the nurses and the houseman working on this ward became involved in the exercise. Although it was obviously impossible for everyone to attend every discussion, a small group managed to meet most days for half an hour or so to share knowledge and ideas about pain management. The general level of interest and concern was raised.

At the end of this time the sister decided that it would be useful to examine the effect of this effort on the pain suffered by their patients. As she wanted to compare these results with the earlier ones she had to think about controlling any other variables which might alter the findings. Although a few of the student nurses on the ward had changed, there had been no major changes in staffing in the period since the first data collection. There were no factors such as bank holidays or surgeon's holidays occurring which might alter the characteristics of the patients admitted.

If possible she wanted to have patients who were as similar as possible to those studied on the first occasion; of about the same age and having the same operation. This could be very difficult to achieve within a reasonable time span. However, they could group the patients into age ranges:

    35–50 (there were no patients younger than 35)
    51–65
    66–75
    76 and over

As patients were admitted to the ward, they were compared with those in the first group and when a patient could be matched for age group and was having the same or a similar operation to his 'twin' he was asked if he would take part in the study. When each patient in the first group had been paired and the data collected, the study was terminated. This took about three and a half weeks. The results obtained were as follows.

Patient	Score
Q	10
R	8
S	11
T	7
U	15
V	8
W	9
X	12
Y	10
Z	9
	99

These results gave a mean of 9.9 over the eight occasions, giving an average of 1.24 per occasion, or just slightly more than a 'just noticeable' degree of pain.

These results clearly show a marked reduction in the pain scores obtained and everyone was pleased with this result. This study was small and the results cannot be generalised beyond this ward. The use of a statistical test is not necessary to demonstrate the result of the 4 week study and thinking among the staff. However, if the sister had decided to carry out a statistical test to check whether these results were statistically significant, the Mann–Whitney U test would have been the appropriate one to use.

Conclusion

We hope that these three small scale examples have demonstrated that the research approach need not be synonymous with complexity and can be quickly and easily used. The statistical analysis can be elementary, for example, the calculation of percentages, although a series of more sophisticated but not difficult statistical techniques have been described in earlier chapters. Statistical analysis has no value, of itself. It is simply a means to an end, so if your research question can be answered through the calculation of a few percentages, so much the better!

A good piece of research, however small, will generally raise as many questions as it answers. Most research studies end with a statement of further research that now needs to be done. The cynics would incline to the view that this is simply a demonstration of researchers keeping themselves in work! As Fletcher Knebel wrote in 1962: 'It is now proved beyond doubt that smoking is one of the leading causes of statistics' (*Concise Oxford Dictionary of Quotations*, 1982). It is nonetheless the case that successful research generates more research and the research process can prove addictive if frustrating.

Mark Pattison (1813–1884), a renowned academic wrote that 'in research, the horizon recedes as we advance, and it is no nearer at sixty than it was at twenty. As the power of endurance weakens with age, the urgency of the pursuit grows more intense . . . and research is always incomplete' (*Concise Oxford Dictionary of Quotations*, 1962). We hope that the readers of this book will now feel some urgency of pursuit in carrying out research, and we look forward to a stock of sixty-year-old nurse researchers creating a manpower problem for the future! Some one no doubt will want to research the problem!

Appendix

The following tables have been adapted from Neave (1981) and Siegel (1956).

Table 1 The student t distribution two-tailed test.

Degrees of freedom	Level of significance 5%	Degrees of freedom	Level of significance 5%
1	12.7062	31	2.0395
2	4.3027	32	2.0369
3	3.1824	33	2.0345
4	2.7764	34	2.0322
5	2.5706	35	2.0301
6	2.4469	36	2.0281
7	2.3646	37	2.0262
8	2.3060	38	2.0244
9	2.2622	39	2.0227
10	2.2281	40	2.0211
11	2.2010	42	2.0181
12	2.1788	44	2.0154
13	2.1604	46	2.0129
14	2.1448	48	2.0106
15	2.1314	50	2.0040
16	2.1199	55	2.0040
17	2.1098	60	2.0003
18	2.1009	65	1.9971
19	2.0930	70	1.9944
20	2.0860	75	1.9921
21	2.0796	80	1.9901
22	2.0739	85	1.9883
23	2.0687	90	1.9867
24	2.0639	95	1.9853
25	2.0595	100	1.9840
26	2.0555	125	1.9791
27	2.0518	150	1.9759
28	2.0484	175	1.9736
29	2.0452	200	1.9719
30	2.0423	∞	1.9600

[N.B. Critical values when testing null hypothesis μ = k against the alternative hypothesis $\mu \neq$ k (two-tailed test).]

Table 2 The student t distribution one-tailed test.

Degrees of freedom	Level of significance 5%	Degrees of freedom	Level of significance 5%
1	6.3138	31	1.6955
2	2.9200	32	1.6939
3	2.3534	33	1.6924
4	2.1318	34	1.6909
5	2.0150	35	1.6896
6	1.9432	36	1.6883
7	1.8946	37	1.6871
8	1.8595	38	1.6860
9	1.8331	39	1.6849
10	1.8125	40	1.6839
11	1.7959	42	1.6820
12	1.7823	44	1.6802
13	1.7709	46	1.6787
14	1.7613	48	1.6759
15	1.7531	50	1.6759
16	1.7459	55	1.6730
17	1.7396	60	1.6706
18	1.7341	65	1.6686
19	1.7291	70	1.6669
20	1.7247	75	1.6654
21	1.7207	80	1.6641
22	1.7171	85	1.6630
23	1.7139	90	1.6620
24	1.7109	95	1.6611
25	1.7081	100	1.6602
26	1.7056	125	1.6571
27	1.7033	150	1.6551
28	1.7011	175	1.6536
29	1.6991	200	1.6525
30	1.6973	∞	1.6449

[N.B. Critical values when testing null hypothesis $\mu = k$ against the alternative hypothesis $\mu > k$ or $\mu < k$ (one-tailed test).]

Table 3 Critical values of d in the Kolmogorov–Smirnov one-sample test.

Sample size	Level of significance for d 5%	Sample size	Level of significance for d 5%
1	.975	16	.328
2	.842	17	.318
3	.708	18	.309
4	.624	19	.301
5	.565	20	.294
6	.521	25	.27
7	.486	30	·.24
8	.457	35	.23
9	.432	Over 35	1.36
10	.410		
11	.391		
12	.375		
13	.361		
14	.349		
15	.338		

Table 4 Critical values for the chi-squared test.

Degrees of freedom	Level of significance 5%	Degrees of freedom	Level of significance 5%
1	3.841	26	38.885
2	5.991	27	40.113
3	7.815	28	41.337
4	9.488	29	42.557
5	11.070	30	43.773
6	12.592	31	44.985
7	14.967	32	46.194
8	15.507	33	47.400
9	16.919	34	48.602
10	18.307	35	49.802
11	19.675	36	50.998
12	21.026	37	55.668
13	22.685	38	53.384
14	23.685	39	54.572
15	24.996	40	55.758
16	26.296	45	61.656
17	27.587	50	67.505
18	28.869	60	79.082
19	30.144	70	90.531
20	31.410	80	101.88
21	32.671	90	113.15
22	33.924	100	124.34
23	35.172	120	146.57
24	36.415	150	179.58
25	37.652	200	233.99

Table 5 Critical values for the Wilcoxon test

Degrees of freedom	Level of significance 5%	Degrees of freedom	Level of significance 5%
1	–	46	361
2	–	47	378
3	–	48	396
4	–	49	415
5	–	50	434
6	0	51	453
7	2	52	473
8	3	53	494
9	5	54	514
10	8	55	536
11	10	56	557
12	13	57	579
13	17	58	602
14	21	59	625
15	25	60	648
16	29	61	672
17	34	62	697
18	40	63	721
19	46	64	747
20	52	65	772
21	58	66	798
22	65	67	825
23	73	68	852
24	81	69	879
25	89	70	907
26	98	71	936
27	107	72	964
28	116	73	994
29	126	74	1023
30	137	75	1053
31	147	76	1084
32	159	77	1115
33	170	78	1147
34	182	79	1179
35	195	80	1211
36	208	81	1244
37	221	82	1277
38	235	83	1311
39	249	84	1345
40	264	85	1380
41	279	86	1415
42	294	87	1451
43	310	88	1487
44	327	89	1523
45	343	90	1560

Table 5 cont'd

Degrees of freedom	Level of significance 5%	Degrees of freedom	Level of significance 5%
91	1676	96	1791
92	1635	97	1832
93	1674	98	1872
94	1712	99	1913
95	1752	100	1955

Table 6 Critical values for the Mann–Whitney U test

Degrees of freedom for two samples (size n_1 and n_2)		Level of signficance 5%	Degrees of freedom for two samples (size n_1 and n_2)		Level of significance 5%
2	2	–	3	23	9
2	3	–	3	24	10
2	4	–	3	25	10
2	5	–			
2	6	–	4	4	0
2	7	–	4	5	1
2	8	0	4	6	2
2	9	0	4	7	3
2	10	0	4	8	4
2	11	0	4	9	4
2	12	1	4	10	5
2	13	1	4	11	6
2	14	1	4	12	7
2	15	1	4	13	8
2	16	1	4	14	9
2	17	2	4	15	10
2	18	2	4	16	11
2	19	2	4	17	11
2	20	2	4	18	12
2	21	3	4	19	13
2	22	3	4	20	14
2	23	3	4	21	15
2	24	3	4	22	16
2	25	3	4	23	17
			4	24	17
3	3	–	4	25	18
3	4	–			
3	5	0	5	5	2
3	6	1	5	6	3
3	7	1	5	7	5
3	8	2	5	8	6
3	9	2	5	9	7
3	10	3	5	10	8
3	11	3	5	11	9
3	12	4	5	12	11
3	13	4	5	13	12
3	14	5	5	14	13
3	15	5	5	15	14
3	16	6	5	16	15
3	17	6	5	17	17
3	18	7	5	18	18
3	19	7	5	19	19
3	20	8	5	20	20
3	21	8	5	21	22
3	22	9	5	22	23

Table 6 cont'd

Degrees of freedom for two samples (size n_1 and n_2)		Level of signficance 5%	Degrees of freedom for two samples (size n_1 and n_2)		Level of significance 5%
5	23	24	8	10	17
5	24	25	8	11	19
5	25	27	8	12	22
			8	13	24
6	6	5	8	14	26
6	7	6	8	15	29
6	8	8	8	16	31
6	9	10	8	17	34
6	10	11	8	18	36
6	11	13	8	19	38
6	12	14	8	20	41
6	13	16	8	21	43
6	14	17	8	22	45
6	15	19	8	23	48
6	16	21	8	24	50
6	17	22	8	25	53
6	18	24			
6	19	25	9	9	17
6	20	27	9	10	20
6	21	29	9	11	23
6	22	30	9	12	26
6	23	32	9	13	28
6	24	33	9	14	31
6	25	35	9	15	34
			9	16	37
7	7	8	9	17	39
7	8	10	9	18	42
7	9	12	9	19	45
7	10	14	9	20	48
7	11	16	9	21	50
7	12	18	9	22	53
7	13	20	9	23	56
7	14	22	9	24	59
7	15	24	9	25	62
7	16	26			
7	17	28	10	10	23
7	18	30	10	11	26
7	19	32	10	12	29
7	20	34	10	13	33
7	21	36	10	14	36
7	22	38	10	15	39
7	23	40	10	16	42
7	24	42	10	17	45
7	25	44	10	18	48
			10	19	52
8	8	13	10	20	55
8	9	15			

Table 6 cont'd

Degrees of freedom for two samples (size n_1 and n_2).		Level of signficance 5%	Degrees of freedom for two samples (size n_1 and n_2)		Level of significance 5%
10	20	55	13	21	80
10	21	58	13	22	85
10	22	61	13	23	89
10	23	64	13	24	94
10	24	67	13	25	98
10	25	71	14	14	55
11	11	30	14	15	59
11	12	33	14	16	64
11	13	37	14	17	69
11	14	40	14	18	74
11	15	44	14	19	78
11	16	47	14	20	83
11	17	51	14	21	88
11	18	55	14	22	93
11	19	58	14	23	98
11	20	62	14	24	102
11	21	65	14	25	107
11	22	69	15	15	64
11	23	73	15	16	70
11	24	76	15	17	75
11	25	80	15	18	80
12	12	37	15	19	85
12	13	41	15	20	90
12	14	45	15	21	96
12	15	49	15	22	101
12	16	53	15	23	106
12	17	57	15	24	111
12	18	61	15	25	117
12	19	65	16	16	75
12	20	69	16	17	81
12	21	73	16	18	86
12	22	77	16	19	92
12	23	81	16	20	98
12	24	85	16	21	103
12	25	89	16	22	109
13	13	45	16	23	115
13	14	50	16	24	120
13	15	54	16	25	126
13	16	59	17	17	87
13	17	63	17	18	93
13	18	67	17	19	99
13	19	72	17	20	105
13	20	76			

Table 6 cont'd

Degrees of freedom for two samples (size n_1 and n_2)		Level of signficance 5%	Degrees of freedom for two samples (size n_1 and n_2)		Level of significance 5%
17	21	111	25	25	211
17	22	117			
17	23	123	26	26	230
17	24	129	27	27	250
17	25	135			
			28	28	272
18	18	99			
18	19	106	29	29	294
18	20	112	30	30	317
18	21	119			
18	22	125	31	31	341
18	23	132	32	32	365
18	24	138			
18	25	145	33	33	391
19	19	113	34	32	418
19	20	119	35	35	445
19	21	126			
19	22	133	36	36	473
19	23	140	37	37	503
19	24	147			
19	25	154	38	38	533
20	20	127	39	39	564
20	21	134	40	40	596
20	22	141			
20	23	149	41	41	628
20	24	156	42	42	662
20	25	163			
			43	43	697
21	21	142	44	44	732
21	22	150			
21	23	157	45	45	769
21	24	165	46	46	806
21	25	173			
			47	47	845
22	22	158	48	48	884
22	23	166			
22	24	174	49	49	924
22	25	182	50	50	965
23	23	175			
23	24	183			
23	25	192			
24	24	192			
24	25	201			

Table 7 Critical values for the Spearman rank correlation coefficient

Degrees of freedom	Level of significance 5%	Degrees of freedom	Level of significance 5%
1	–	46	0.2913
2	–	47	0.2880
3	–	48	0.2850
4	–	49	0.2820
5	1.0000	50	0.2791
6	0.8857	51	0.2764
7	0.7857	52	0.2736
8	0.7381	53	0.2710
9	0.7000	54	0.2685
10	0.6485	55	0.2659
11	0.6182	56	0.2636
12	0.5874	57	0.2612
13	0.5604	58	0.2589
14	0.5385	59	0.2567
15	0.5214	60	0.2545
16	0.5029	61	0.2524
17	0.4877	62	0.2503
18	0.4716	63	0.2483
19	0.4596	64	0.2463
20	0.4466	65	0.2444
21	0.4364	66	0.2425
22	0.4252	67	0.2407
23	0.4160	68	0.2229
24	0.4070	69	0.2372
25	0.3977	70	0.2354
26	0.3901	71	0.2337
27	0.3828	72	0.2321
28	0.3755	73	0.2305
29	0.3685	74	0.2289
30	0.3624	75	0.2274
31	0.3560	76	0.2259
32	0.3504	77	0.2244
33	0.3449	78	0.2229
34	0.3396	79	0.2215
35	0.3347	80	0.2201
36	0.3300	82	0.2174
37	0.3253	84	0.2147
38	0.3209	86	0.2122
39	0.3168	88	0.2097
40	0.3128	90	0.2074
41	0.3087	92	0.2051
42	0.3051	94	0.2029
43	0.3014	96	0.2008
44	0.2978	98	0.1987
45	0.2945	100	0.1967

References

Boore, J. (1978). *Prescription for Recovery*. Royal College of Nursing, London.

Briggs Report (1972). Report of the Committee on Nursing. Cmnd 115. HMSO, London.

Concise Oxford Dictionary of Quotations (1982). Oxford University Press, Oxford.

Cochrane, W. (1977). *Sampling Techniques*, 3rd edition, John Wiley & Sons, London.

Cook, S. W. (1976). Ethical Issues in the Conduct of Research in Social Relations. In *Research Methods in Social Relations*. C. Selltiz, L. Wrightsman and S. W. Cook (eds). Holt–Saunders International Editions.

de Dombal, F. T., Leaper, D. J., Horrocks, J. C., Staniland, J. R., McCann, A. P. (1974). Human and Computer-Aided Diagnosis of Abdominal Pain: Further Report with Emphasis on Performance of Clinicians. *British Medical Journal*, **1**, 376–80.

Hayward, J. (1975). *Information – a prescription against pain*. Royal College of Nursing, London.

Huff, D. (1954). *How to Lie with Statistics*. Gollancz, London.

McCaffery, M. (1979). *Nursing the Patient in Pain* (adapted for the UK by B. Sofaer). Harper & Row, London.

Moser, C. and Kalton, G. (1972). *Survey Methods in Social Investigation*. Heinemann, London.

Neave, H. (1981). *Elementary Statistics Tables for all users of statistical techniques*. George Allen & Unwin, London.

Pearson, K. (1924). *The Life, Letters and Labours of Francis Galton*, Vol. ii, Ch. xiii, Sect. i. Cambridge University Press, Cambridge.

Reid, N. (1986). *Wards in Chancery? Nurse Training in the Clinical Area*. Royal College of Nursing, London.

Reid, N. G. and Melaugh, M. (1987). Nurse Hours Per Patient: A Method for Monitoring and Explaining Staffing Levels. *International Journal of Nursing Studies*, **24**(1), 1–14.

Siegel, S. (1956). *Nonparametric Statistics for the Behavioural Sciences*. McGraw-Hill, Kogakusha Ltd.

Index